BETTER BODY
WANNABE

Better Body **Wannabe**

*12 Top Trainers Reveal the Real Skinny on
Eating and Exercising for a
More Healthy, Happy, and Fit YOU*

TIFFANY YOUNGREN

Founder of Transfer of Health

TRANSFER OF HEALTH, LLC
TransferofHealth.com

First Printing, 2014

ISBN: 0615929818
ISBN-13: 978-0-615-92981-1

Transfer of Health, LLC

28 Shane Ridge Road

Columbus, MT 59019

www.TransferofHealth.com

For my inspiring husband, Duane,
and my amazing kids,
Alex, Devin, and Miranda –
keep letting your lights shine.

To my fellow wannabes:
You can – and will – do it!
This is your time.

Table of Contents

Introduction

I can already hear you now: "Oh no, not another diet book!" And yet, here you are reading another diet book! But it's not just another diet book; it's not just another anything. Above all, this book is an opportunity for you to take stock of your health, find out where you are and what you want to do, and then do it.

But you won't be alone; not this time. First, let me introduce myself. My name is Tiffany Youngren, and I run TransferofHealth.com. Not long ago, I was a lot like you. I basically ate what I wanted when I wanted, and I didn't think much about alternative medicine. I went to the doctor when I was sick and exercised when I felt like it; you know the drill.

Then my husband, Duane, fell and experienced excruciating back pain that never quite went away. After following the usual route of going to traditional doctors, who merely prescribed pills, we watched his health spiral dangerously out of control. Then we were given the name of a local naturopath and, well, the rest is history.

Health became a driving concern for my husband and me, so much so that I set about starting a new business, TransferofHealth.com, and began interviewing health experts around the country for the best ways to achieve a better body!

And that's where you come in. *Better Body Wannabe* is NOT another diet book. In fact, it's not a diet book at all. It's a sampling, I would say, of what some of today's brightest, finest, most dedicated and most helpful health experts have to say about what you eat, how you move, and why achieving a healthy weight is the one investment we can all afford to make—and can't afford *not* to make!

What This Book Is About

- *Going from being a better body wannabe to, "Yeah, baby!"*

- *Making simple changes that stick*

- *Gathering information from many sources*

- *Finding ways to make wellness affordable*

- *Adopting a can-do attitude*

- *Valuing the opinions of professionals who value the opinions of other professionals*

- *Eating junk food sometimes, especially if it means spending time with our friends, but trying to prepare and plan well so that is rarely necessary.*

What This Book Is NOT About

- *Judging the shortcomings of a sincere effort*

- *Letting food become the boss of our lives. Whether it*

dictates that we eat poorly or it pulls at our tendency to obsess about eating perfectly, food is NOT the boss. The people around us are far more important than the food we eat.

Meet the Top 12 Trainers

I have been so fortunate in finding twelve elite health experts, authors, bloggers, and personal trainers to interview for this groundbreaking book. They are knockout gorgeous on the outside and beautiful on the inside, and they represent a generational spectrum as they generously offer all they know about how to live life to its fullest. This is an eclectic group of people who are friendly, helpful, and kind. I'm just sure you'll find each of them informative as you zero in on a few who you specifically connect with.

So, why does it matter what *these* twelve trainers have to say? Well, if you're like me, you don't want to be told what to do, but prefer encouragement through stories from the experiences of a wide range of people, especially professional people.

This very diverse group of trainers has influenced millions of people like you and me who are struggling to get fit one day at a time, and each has a unique vantage point.

As you read this book, you will reap the benefits of several world-renowned trainers, including the founder of iBodyFit. com and the humble and heroic Gilad Janklowicz, the host of everyone's favorite and long-running *Bodies in Motion* series. You will be encouraged by the author of *Workouts for Dummies* and the star of *Buns of Steel*. You will be amazed at the breadth of knowledge that each of these personal trainers shares with you individually and collectively in *Better Body Wannabe*.

For now, here are the 12 trainers that will finally help you achieve your better body:

Adriana Martin

As the author of *The Pregnancy Weight Book*, featured trainer on Univision's morning show *Tu Desayuno Alegre*, and reality show trainer for *The Balancing Act* on Lifetime Television, Adriana has created an innovative approach to helping clients and viewers achieve their health and fitness goals through all the seasons of life and despite the time constraints of motherhood. In addition to being a talented trainer who balances her busy schedule with a thriving family life, Adriana is a dynamic, driven, and very talented businesswoman with a magnetic sense of passion and positivity.

Allyson Shumate

Ally got started as a personal trainer part-time in 2006 after working as a project manager on major capital construction projects for over twenty years. Four years later, Ally opened her own studio in Tennessee and now coaches full time. Ally's goal is to get people hooked on exercise and to realize that we don't need a gym or expensive equipment to get fit and enjoy an active lifestyle.

Donovan Green

With over twelve years of professional experience, Donovan is a specialist in muscle confusion. He fuses exercises ranging from sports conditioning to yoga, all within one session. Donovan has a diverse list of clients, including celebrities such as Dr. Oz, who are passionate about maintaining their physical appearance and devoted to his unique style of training. Donovan's positive attitude, his energy, and his "why not?" mentality empower his clients with the sense of greatness needed to attain their unique and specific goals. He strongly believes that procrastination is the key to failure.

Ashley Borden

Ashley is an author, exercise guru, and fitness and lifestyle consultant to several world-class athletes and some of Hollywood's most recognizable faces. Her clients include Christina Aguilera, Natasha Bedingfield, Mandy Moore, Ryan Gosling, Nick Swisher of the New York Yankees, and UFC champion Matt Hughes. She has been recognized by publications such as *Elle* Japan, *Harper's Bazaar* Russia, *Who* Australia, and London's *NOW* magazine. In addition, she has been a featured expert on the Today Show, Rachael Ray, Discovery Health, the Tyra Banks Show, MTV, VH1, E! Entertainment, and more. Ashley is a powerhouse whose drive and unrelenting pursuit of excellence is highly motivating and encouraging.

David Vaughan

David is the CEO of Forget the Gym in Las Vegas. Their mission is to provide safe, high-quality fitness training for the residents of Las Vegas. Since 2005, David has worked with several local professional athletes, entrepreneurs, poker pros, news personalities, entertainers such as Barry Manilow, and the cast of "The Phantom of the Opera." He earned a bachelor of science degree in exercise science, and holds several certifications in strength training, conditioning, and personal training, including MMA strength and conditioning. David's work speaks to his clients' core motivators. Where else but in Vegas can people (legally) place bets on their own fitness goals?

Franklin Antoian

Franklin is the founder of iBodyFit.com, which offers free and premium online workouts, exercise videos, yoga, pilates, Vlogs (video blogs), and more! He is an American Council on Exercise certified personal trainer, as well as a fitness writer and expert for ManageMyLife.com. In 2013, Franklin was featured as one of *Shape* magazine's Top 50 Hottest Trainers in America. He is a mover and shaker in today's Internet and social media-driven fitness programs.

Gilad Janklowicz

Gilad is one of the world's most popular fitness personalities. He has trained celebrities such as Arnold Schwarzenegger, Jack LaLanne, and quarterback Joe Theismann—all of whom appeared on his television program, "Bodies in Motion," shot in the beautiful Hawaiian Islands. As a pioneer in the fitness industry who was elected into the Fitness Hall of Fame, Gilad has helped millions to stay fit with his popular TV fitness shows "Basic Training, the Workout" and the series "Total Body Sculpt with Gilad." He also offers instructional home fitness DVDs and videos. Gilad's fitness experience is unparalleled, his gentleness mesmerizing, and his humility is ... well ... humbling. I hope you enjoy reading his chapter as much as I enjoyed writing it.

Heather Hodges

"Coach Heather" is passionate about helping adults and kids take charge of their health and wellness through fitness and solid nutrition. She is a CrossFit Trainer and holds certifications in Olympic lifting, kettlebells, CrossFit Gymnastics, movement and mobility, and CrossFit Kids. *Austin Fit Magazine* selected her as one of Austin's Top 10 Fittest Moms in 2010. She is the picture of a busy mom who successfully (and impressively) lives a full family, spiritual, health-centered, and career life.

Kelli Buzzard

Kelli Buzzard is a Beachbody coach in Northwest Washington, and her passion for fitness, nutrition, and overall health has only grown. Kelli is a certified P90X trainer and NESTA-certified fitness nutrition coach. In addition to training people in her home, at local Fit Clubs, and on the Internet, she loves discovering how the human body works and how nutrition plays a role in proper function and physical fitness.

Lindsay Wright

Lindsay runs "Lindsay's List," a healthy living blog, where she shares lists of things that she's working on. There you'll find workouts, recipes, adorable kids, and what she describes as "bad jokes." Her readers love her! Lindsay is an NASM-certified personal trainer, group fitness instructor, #Fitfluential Ambassador, and stay-at-home mom all rolled into one.

Tamilee Webb

You may recognize Tamilee from *Buns of Steel* or her dozen or so videos since then, as a cohost on Discovery's *Fit TV* or host of ESPN's *Body Squad*, or from her four bestselling books, including *Workouts for Dummies*. She has been elected into the prestigious Fitness Hall of Fame. Her knowledge and acquired experience, combined with her contagious energy and effervescent personality, have made her an ideal guest speaker on top-rated television talk shows, including *Entertainment Tonight*, *The Today Show*, *E! Entertainment*, and *The BIG Idea* on CNBC. Tamilee's well-toned body has graced the covers of *Shape Magazine* and *Fitness*. She has been featured in *Fit Magazine*, *Men's Fitness*, *Vogue*, *American Fitness*, and *Billboard*.

Thomas "Doc" Masters

"Doc" is the founder of Flex-Appeal, a premier, accomplished, personal training company he has operated in Orange

County, California with non-athletes in weight loss and fitness, and with the elderly in assisted care facilities. He is a licensed USCG captain and PADI scuba instructor. Doc is a pioneer in the personal training field, and he sets the bar high when it comes to staying fit and active for the long haul.

———

Want more from the trainers? Visit www.TransferofHealth.com regularly to hear audio excerpts from interviews with the trainers. When you hear the passionate professionals speak, you will be inspired to live better right away.

A Few Words about *Better Body Wannabe*

I wrote this book because once upon a time, health, diet, and fitness were like three blind mice that I chased, ignored, chased, ignored, and chased again. I wrote this book because my transformed relationship with all three saved my husband's life, and in the process, turned mine around. I wrote this book because I wish someone had written this book for me way back when.

I believe this is a simple guide told straight from the mouths of some of today's hottest health and fitness experts in a way that very simply but bluntly gives you the basics about what, when, where, why, and, most importantly, how to start living your life the right way, the healthy way, in order to achieve a better body!

Preface

It Ain't Rocket Science
by **Tiffany Youngren**

"Don't judge each day by the harvest you reap
but by the seeds that you plant."
~ Robert Louis Stevenson

Many people say, "I need to lose weight. I can only lose weight if someone tells me exactly what to do." Often I'll hear, "I really need help. Can you help me?" Like many of the trainers, I want to help. The biggest question is this: What does help look like? Does it mean writing out a step-by-step foolproof plan? Have you asked for help? What is it that you want? Do you *really* want someone calling you every day, every week, or every once in a while and holding you accountable? You may think you want that type of help, but it is extremely unlikely that you would enjoy it.

This exact dilemma is what sparked *Better Body Wannabe*. Thinking about the idea that so many of us are wannabes stirred up many questions in my mind that all pointed to one, big, common problem: How can we stop ourselves from sitting around and *thinking* about working out (being a wannabe) and actually find enough drive to *do* something—to take action. Being a wannabe just means that we are procrastinating.

Procrastination has many sneaky disguises. The trainers discuss many of these disguises—they are the excuses they hear us say to avoid working out. Another disguise is what some of us wannabes call planning. If only we had the perfect plan, a schedule, or an accountability program, then we would work out. If you're like me, that perfect plan can be researched, reworked, and rewritten over and over again for days, and even weeks' worth of procrastination (this is akin to analysis paralysis). We also sometimes use the excuse that we need help: if only someone would help me, I would be fit. The truth is that there is no such thing. How does someone help you exercise? Do they call you every day, week, or once in a while? If you go that route, don't ask a friend; before too long, you won't like that person because you'll feel she is a nag that you only want to avoid. You'll be afraid for her to see you eating or enjoying yourself when you really should be working out and eating healthy.

So, here is my recommendation for how to use what you've learned from 12 of my favorite trainers ever. I'm only going to give you four steps, because I agree with the awesome people featured in this book: *Keep it SIMPLE.*

#1: Write your excuses on paper, then shred it. If you really want to change your wannabe ways, write down your excuses on a piece of paper, fold it up, then shred it. Pray that you will be released from those excuses that bound you in the past, and declare yourself free from them forever.

#2: Write your three favorite trainer Tips from *Better Body Wannabe.* Now that procrastination is out of the way, write down three of your favorite tips from the trainers. There are so many tips, but one that resonates is to keep it simple and don't do too much too soon. So, just write down *three improvements* you are going to make, then make them—starting NOW!

#3: Do it. Start today. The waiting is over. Congratulations! Don't make more than one list. Resist the temptation to wait for something that will make the time seem right. Just do those three things—anyone can do three things. Keep it simple.

You will find at the end of this book all the trainer's top 12 lists. Go through them, or reread your favorite chapter to get the back story and motivation of each trainer so that you can really take in those tips.

#4: Repeat. As soon as you nail the first three tips, write down three more and repeat.

If I could encourage you to do one thing that I know would help you to go from being a wannabe straight to having the mindset of "yeah, baby!" it would be this: internalize the idea that you want to make each change to better yourself today. Avoid setting weight loss goals. Stay away from the scale.

I asked every trainer, "If you were the boss of the world, what is one free, simple change you would require people to make?" My answer to that question is this: ditch the obsession with weight loss and embrace health.

What does health mean? I'm talking about looking at you tomorrow and saying, "Wow! Something about you is different. What is it? Your eyes are brighter, and your skin has really good color." Then you would reply, "Well, I slept eight hours, I drank four glasses of water, and I replaced drive-through fast food with homemade fast food." That'll do it. People who make even the smallest changes immediately find themselves thinking more clearly, feeling more rested, and being in a better mood.

As you make more and more changes, you will feel better and better. Guess what? One day, you'll step on the scale and say, "Hey! I lost ten pounds when I wasn't even looking!" That is a great reward, but no greater than feeling good. In no time, you'll notice yourself feeling yucky when you eat food that is harmful, or when you miss a few glasses a water or skip a workout. Now THAT is a great reward: when you exercise and eat great just because you want to.

Nothing in this book is rocket science, but rocket science isn't what we need to go from wannabe to "yeah, baby!" What we need is strategy, motivation, and encouragement to act. I hope this book provides you with all three.

Chapter 1

Fitness as a Family Affair
with **Adriana Martin**

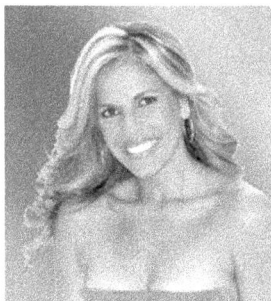

"I really believe in progression when it comes to working out. So you have to learn to crawl before you get up and walk, and you have to be walking really well before you run."
~ **Adriana Martin**

For more than a decade, Adriana Martin has devoted her fitness career to teaching women and their families how to stay fit and fabulous! As the author of *The Pregnancy Weight Book*, Adriana has created an innovative approach to helping modern women achieve their health and fitness goals through all the seasons of life and despite the time constraints of motherhood.

Through her own business and as the fitness contributor for *Tu Desayuno Alegre* on Univision and *The Balancing Act* on Lifetime TV, Adriana has devised creative, fun-filled, and practical methods for women at all stages of life *and* health;

from individual women to moms-to-be, all the way to the entire family.

Adriana's dynamic personality and knowledge make her a sought-after expert for popular English- and Spanish-language television programs and specialized websites including *The Evening News with Katie Couric, South Florida Today Show, Desayuno Alegre, CNN Headline News, Comcast Newsmakers* and WebMD.com, to name just a few.

"Women know the importance of taking care of themselves, but somehow the balance between work, home, family, and personal fulfillment becomes more and more difficult to achieve," explains Martin. "Today, many women find that taking care of themselves is the last thing on their to-do list. This only creates a vicious cycle. Adult obesity is on the rise, and so is childhood obesity. We must do something."

To break the cycle, Adriana teaches that *fitness is a family affair,* and should become a lifestyle where parents need to lead the way! Through her website, educational videos, programs, and seminars, Adriana has created the ultimate resource for people who are seeking practical advice, proven techniques, and energizing motivation.

Adriana considers herself a "health and wellness mompreneur," with her two children keeping her busy and showing her that fitness really can—and should—be a family affair. Adriana is self-employed and has a couple of businesses up and running at the moment, but her main goal is just to find channels to be able to promote health and fitness in her role as a lifestyle ambassador.

One of those distribution channels, she's discovered, is the World Wide Web. Says Adriana, "The Internet is a beautiful way to connect with thousands of people. Some people have described me as an Internet marketer, but I just think that the Internet is my channel, and it's a beautiful one."

One of the things Adriana uses the Internet for is social media, as a way to share her incredible story. But wait, I'll let her tell it herself: "I was born in Venezuela, South America, and my mom—I'm thirty-four years old, so just imagine thirty-four years back; she was a yoga instructor, and she was a vegetarian, and I grew up eating brown rice and not eating meat. It was very different from what it is now.

"Thirty-four years ago, people thought vegetarians were crazy, especially in the small town where I'm from. My mom was a person who did yoga and took care of herself, but it wasn't cool at the time like it is now.

"I remember being seven and thinking, *I really want to eat meat, because if we go to a birthday party and somebody's trying a hotdog, I can't have it*, and *I feel so different from my friends and the other families*.

"I said to my mom, 'I really want to eat it because that will make me blend in and fit in.'

"So my mom said, 'It's your path and you're young, but if you have such a strong conviction about it….' She actually gave me the opportunity to do whatever I wanted.

"My parents were divorced at the time, so I would go to my father's house and have more of a regular type life, and with her it was very, very healthy. I think, at a young age, I got to experience both sides of the spectrum, and when I turned twenty-one, I moved to the United States, and it was about working three jobs and making money and getting very low pay, and working hard, not eating well, and going to fast food places. That was my life at the time. I remember one day just feeling so exhausted and tired, and thinking to myself that I wasn't born like this.

"My mom was the healthiest person I could think of, and I needed to go back to that. That's when everything started, about thirteen years ago. This is one of the reasons why I say to moms, 'You have to lead by example, and you have to be the one.' Because my mom didn't force it upon me.

"She didn't want me to just do it. She allowed me to be who I wanted to be, but it was her example that brought me back, at twenty-something years, to say, 'I want to be more like her.' That's when my whole journey in the fitness industry started."

And what a journey it's been! Now a mother herself, Adriana is in frequent contact with other mothers, other family ambassadors, who want optimal health for their families. Moms are constantly asking her questions such as, "Adriana, how can I get my kids to eat healthy?"

Says Adriana, "A lot of moms get on a healthy pattern, and they research so much about food coloring and what it does, and they try not to eat too much sugar. Sometimes as a mom I understand, because I want the best for my kids, but sometimes it's also allowing them to see you doing the best that you can, but allowing them to have that little bit of freedom and not force healthy food on them so much. Because if you can be the example, sooner or later, they will remember, and they will make healthier choices."

Throughout the course of her career, Adriana has discovered that she enjoys teaching fitness to groups of people, spreading her message to the class *and* the individual. "I've always enjoyed just the group," she explains, "and the whole vibe of having more than one person—just belonging to something like the little friendships that you have when you're in a group setting."

Little by little, course by course, Adriana has what she refers to as a ton of certifications. From being in the first infomercial for Zumba when it came out, to Pilates, to everything in between, Adriana offers her clients a full range of training possibilities.

Having become known as a fitness ambassador, today Adriana specializes in one-on-one instruction, tending to an exclusive list of clients who appreciate her passion and expertise. But what does she do to stay in such great shape?

Surprisingly, Adriana still loves to go to the gym and get instruction from other fitness ambassadors. "What I try to do is just take a little bit of the traditional and the nontraditional, and then always kind of squeeze in a class with an amazing instructor that reminds me of myself when I was younger and was so excited to come in and teach. I just fall in love with these personalities, and that motivation keeps me going."

Perhaps Adriana appreciates the enthusiasm of young trainers so much because it reminds her of her own evolution as a sought-after trainer in her field. She recalls, "Back when I became a fitness instructor, I was teaching twenty-five classes a week—all in different gyms. So I was living in my car and having my food with me for the entire day.

"I would have a cooler, pack my food, and drive from gym to gym, show up and teach. I was so exhausted. I remember somebody said to me 'Hey, they're looking for an instructor at this one gym; do you want to just come try and see?' So I was hired by these people, and then there's the owner, his name's Phil Kaplan. I don't know if you've ever heard of him, but that was the owner of that one gym.

"I remember one day, he looked at me. I don't know if he'll remember this, but he said, 'Wow, you're busy. You are so busy. How do you keep up with everything you do?' I think I needed somebody to tell me, 'Adriana, relax, and see this as a business,' because at the time I was just doing what I loved. And definitely Phil Kaplan—I'm talking about probably ten years ago—from that day, from that first encounter, I became a manager at his gym, and after that we became really, really good friends 'til today."

Learning from mentors and being a mentor must be in Adriana's blood, because she currently is on the Lifetime channel mentoring others in front of millions of people. She explains, "Right now I am doing a reality series called *The Balancing Act* that airs on Lifetime Television. They show four trainers, and one of those four is me. I'm the only female trainer, so it's very interesting because I get to go up against three guys that are amazing as well. Each one of us got a person [to train], and my person, her name's Rosa, she was two hundred forty-eight pounds. She was fifty-one years old, and she was in pre-menopause, and she was having a lot of health issues with her blood pressure and triglycerides. Everything was off the charts in a negative way.

"When I got her, and they told me, 'This is the person you're going to be working out with for the next six months,' I said, 'Wow, I do have my work cut out for me, because it's going to be a lot of work.' Somebody who has reached two hundred forty-eight pounds has forgotten what it means to eat healthy, right? Or maybe they didn't even know what it was. Maybe they've been on yo-yo dieting for their entire lives, and they don't know what it is to eat healthy. So that's why I knew it was going to be a little bit of a challenge. But the good news is that now she's lost fifty pounds. She's doing great. Her health is awesome, and she's definitely my demographic. I think that my goal is really to inspire people who are not fit and healthy."

That's what's so inspiring about Adriana and many of the other trainers profiled in this book: their decision to go into a field where their job description is to motivate others.

So, how can Adriana motivate you? Let me count the ways—a dozen ways, in fact! Here are Adriana's top 12 tips for motivating you to your *more healthy, happy, and fit YOU.*

Top 12 Tips from Adriana

#1: Find a workout that's right for you! My type of clientele is not the clientele that you typically find at the gym. They don't necessarily love exercising. So my first goal is not to give them a super strong, "kick butt" type workout. It's actually a workout that's going to make them feel better and empowered and that's going to boost their endorphins so that they're going to say, "Wow! I feel great. I want to come back."

#2: Timing is everything. I really believe in progression when it comes to working out. So you have to learn to crawl before you get up and walk, and you have to be walking really well before you run. I always put people on a mild workout at the beginning so that they feel accomplished, so that they feel that they are good at what they're doing, and so that they can see the benefit of everything. With Rosa, to give you a very specific example, I got her to sit down on the floor the first day, to get her on the mat. She had such a hard time getting up, and she hated it. She felt embarrassed toward me. She felt embarrassed with herself that she had such a hard time getting up from the floor. So I decided to make a workout that forced her to squat and pick things up from the floor, and to have to mimic that motion of sitting down and getting up so that now she's a pro at it. You should see her! She's lost fifty pounds, and that makes her feel so accomplished. It means so much more to her than just the weight loss, because not only is she fifty pounds lighter, but now she can get on the floor and play with her kids. That's the actual benefit. This is why we need to exercise—not just to look good, but to be better at our lives.

#3: Less is more. What's important to you? What do you want to accomplish in your physical body, in your emotional being, and in your personal life? If I don't know what is important to a particular client, when she shows up, I say, "I'm a trainer; I have to do this." I do a really good workout with her because she has to feel the burn tomorrow, and right now, so she will hire me again." And then I give her ten pushups and fifty sit-ups, and I keep her doing a workout that she's constantly, for an entire session, thinking, *I am so bad at this. I am terrible. I can't do it. This is the reason why I don't work out.* Then it doesn't matter how hard I work her. It was a total failure, and it wasn't a successful training. So that's why sometimes less is more. You never arrive. You always live— until you don't live. So the healthy journey needs to be a lifestyle forever.

#4: Money shouldn't be an obstacle. Your body doesn't know the difference between being at the gym, being at home, being at the park, or being at your neighbor's house. So if you're budgeting, don't feel that you have to join the gym to get in shape, because your body doesn't really know the difference. A squat is a squat, at the gym or at home.

#5: Invest in food! By food I mean whole food, not supplements. Invest it in fruits, vegetables, and healthy protein. But invest the most amount of your budget on your food. The rest, the workout, you can do for free (see above tip!).

#6: Have a sustainable workout. You have to really know why you're doing it, and you have to really want it. Because, I'll tell you what I run away from: I've had people who want to hire me, and they tell me, "Can you make me lose weight? Can you do it? Will you do it? Will you make me lose weight?" And that's when I say, "No, I can't even work with you. That's the wrong mindset, because nobody can make you do anything." You can buy my program for $16.99, and it's an amazing program. I put it together. I gave it my all. And all that information is awesome, but I can't jump out of a picture and make you do anything. So it has to come from your desire to change. Your desire to change and your commitment need to be with yourself. It's not because of your husband; it's not because of your children; it's not because of your friends. It's because of who you are as a person. Do you want to walk through your life feeling like you've accomplished and lived the best way that you possibly can? Or do you always want to be that type of person who wishes that they can have a better body or better health or better "this"? So the mindset comes from being committed one hundred percent. The answer should always be, "No, I'm committed one hundred ten percent. I'm committed one hundred twenty percent. I have to get this going." Once you really know that you want to get up every day and do this, I would say the sustainable workout is Monday, Wednesday, Friday. It could be Tuesday, Thursday, and Saturday, but just leave one day in between. There has to be resistance training. So whether you do it at the gym with machines, or you do it to one of my programs with dumbbells, or to somebody else's program with bands, or you use your own body weight, your muscles have to be trained to work against resistance. Then the other days you have to train what I say is the most important muscle in your body, which is the heart, and do cardiovascular activities.

#7: Have realistic expectations. When a woman wore a size 6 ten years ago, and now she's a size 14, and she wants to get back into a size 6 in six months, and it took her six years to get to where she's at now, it's frustrating. We have that society where instant gratification is so important. We want to see things right away. That's why it's important to set small goals and celebrate each one of those goals so that you stay motivated, and you keep going.

#8: Build a memory bank instead of an excuse bank! What I recommend is, when you have an amazing workout, take the time to close your eyes and replay that memory. One day, you go to a class, and you feel like you can take on the world. Your endorphins are kicking in, and you're super happy. You're on a natural high. Close your eyes and save that feeling. Next time you feel like not going to the gym, go and find that memory; remember how amazing it feels after you're done working out. Then just get up from your chair and get moving.

#9: Do it for more than your looks! The people who actually stay on a healthy lifestyle do it because of the feelings. It's like you eat well, you exercise, you feel better. You want life to be better. You treat others better. Don't do it because of the way you want to look.

#10: Stop making excuses. We think everybody blames the same thing: lack of time. That's a very popular one. I think that takes care of everything else, because all the other excuses are based on time—and money.

#11: Forget your genetics. Women look at their moms and their sisters and their aunts and think that because their bodies are a certain way, then they have to look like that also. It's a "we're all built this way" kind of deal. They fail to realize that they all have the same patterns for life. They have the same eating patterns; they have the same activity patterns, and therefore they kind of all fall into that category. You don't have to be a victim of your metabolism or your genetics. You can actually do something about it.

#12: Believe in yourself! Because when you don't believe, and you've never had anybody coach you on how to achieve things, or how to have the mindset you need in order to get things done, then you don't believe that you can do it. What the brain does is find the excuses. It finds the reasons why I can't do it, but the true reason is that I don't even know where to begin. So that's what I really think about. Anybody who wants to do something can do it. They will find a way to do it. If you don't even think that you can, then that's it.

Thanks, Adriana, for helping us understand what makes you tick, and for offering us a peek into one of your training sessions!

Chapter 2

Get Rid of Your Excuses
with **Allyson Shumate**

"People are afraid they're not going to be successful, afraid that they won't be able to keep it up. I think a lot of people put weight on almost as if it's a coat of armor that's protecting them from something."
~ Ally Shumate

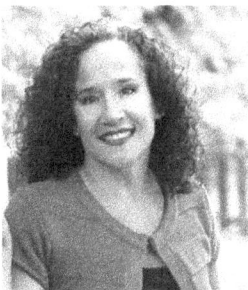

Allyson "Ally" Shumate's background in fitness is unique because she comes from the corporate world as opposed to the traditional "gym rat" route. Says Ally, "I was a project manager on major capital construction projects for more than twenty years, and I got started doing this part-time in 2006. Last year I opened my own studio, and now I'm doing it full time.

Ally's company, AllyFitness, offers results-oriented programs. Whether you are just getting started or need to kick it up a notch, AllyFitness has the tools and flexibility you need to reach your fitness goals. The programs focus on strength training to build muscle to boost your resting metabolism.

Ally's philosophy is known as metabolic training, which is proven to build muscle, blast fat, and get results. This is a no-nonsense approach that gets you fit without spending count-less hours at the gym.

Ally has a proven track record of getting people get fit who never thought they could be. That's because Ally believes that "overcoming mental blocks is the first step in achieving the goal of an active lifestyle."

Ally also has a unique approach in that she focuses on strength and metabolic training as opposed to the cardio rou-tines that make up so much of what so many other personal trainers teach.

Ally explains why her approach is so unique, and the almost accidental way she stumbled across it. "I had to quit running several years ago because of my feet, and that's when I started getting into strength training. That's when I started noticing the biggest changes to my body."

Like many personal trainers interviewed for this book, Ally has a special mentor in the fitness world. Hers is Rachel Cosgrove. Ally explains, "I had a very stressful, demanding job. I used to run about an hour a day, and that was kind of how I stayed in shape.

"And then when I got plantar fasciitis in both feet, I had to quit. I thought, *Oh, my gosh, what am I going to do to man-age my stress and keep my weight managed when I can hardly even walk my dog?*

"I had dumbbells, and so I went online and bought some magazines and I started doing total body strength training three days a week, on Monday, Wednesday, and Friday, like a circuit. After about six weeks, I dropped a jeans size.

"I was working out four or five hours less per week, and my feet didn't hurt! So, I started doing a lot of research on how building the muscle increases your metabolism, and how over time—even when you're at rest—the more intense metabolic workouts where you're working your whole body three days a week are just so much more efficient.

"Rachel Cosgrove has written a good bit about that, so I started doing a lot of research and reading a lot of what she's put out there. That's the philosophy that I follow."

Like most of us, Ally struggled with a day job and trying to stay in shape. "I guess I was like everybody else," she says. "I would do really good for a while, and then life would kind of get in the way and take over. I would get off it for a while, and then try to get back into it. I always had a hard time being able to do it consistently.

"Then once I could just do it three days a week and not have to feel like I had to spend an hour every day, I kind of figured it out. I really want to share this with other women, because I think women struggle more than anybody else."

It was that drive to help other women find self-control and to realize their fitness goals that inspired Ally to open her own gym. "That's kind of why I decided to get into this business," she explains, "to try to help women mostly. I think my main demographic is women between the ages of fifty and sixty. Of course I have some younger clients, and I have some men, but I train mostly middle-aged women."

Ally is proud of how she's turned her own life around as well as the lives of many of her clients. She says, "I have several women who came to me after they were diagnosed with osteopenia and really needed to get the strength training in. I've had several of them get their diagnosis reversed after working out here."

One woman in particular is an inspiration to Ally. "I have one lady who couldn't even do a lunge when she started, and now she's one of my star clients, and she does pushups on her toes. It's just amazing how strong they get."

Ally uses what she calls a metabolic workout, or a total body workout, which she describes as "a high-intensity work period with short rest periods. We work all muscle groups each time. So, instead of working legs one day and back one day and biceps one day, we're working it all each day. So, over the course of the week you're getting more load on those muscles to create the most amount of change, and that's the way we really get rid of the fat. You're building muscle and you're getting rid of the fat."

Unlike many personal trainers, Ally is dead set against gauging success in terms of the scale. She explains, "I don't like people to weigh. When people come here, we do before and after measurements. Like our saying, the scale lies, but the jeans don't."

Ally is full of such great truisms, and when I asked her if she could provide readers with handy ways to reach their fitness goals without sacrificing the other areas of their life, she was quick to comply.

So now, here are Ally's top 12 fitness, nutrition, health, and general life tips for reaching your *more healthy, happy, and fit YOU.*

Top 12 Tips from Ally

#1: Balance your cardio. People focus too much on cardio. I think that doing the weights, the resistance training, is what's going to change your body. I think most people focus too much on cardio, and they feel like they have to do it for at least an hour, or else it doesn't matter.

#2: Lose your all-or-nothing mentality. If you've only got twenty minutes, do something. A lot of people say, "I don't have the time; I can't do it." Well, even if you've only got twenty minutes, if you do something, it's a lot better than doing nothing. It doesn't have to be all or nothing. It can be a little bit here, a little bit there, especially if you haven't been active in a long time.

#3: Don't let your life get in the way. Life gets in the way. People get busy with their job and their family, and then they have it in their mind that it's got to be something they have to commit to for an hour every day, or at least every other day, and it seems an insurmountable task at that time in their life.

#4: Little things can really add up. Something is better than nothing. I think people just let exercise overwhelm them because they have in their mind that it's so much bigger than it needs to be. Whereas, if they could take a walk for twenty minutes at lunchtime, they would feel better.

#5: Get rid of the fear. People are afraid they're not going to be successful; they're afraid that they won't be able to keep it up. I think a lot of people put weight on almost as if it's a coat of armor that's protecting them from something.

#6: Walk more. When we were kids, we walked to school. We rode our bikes all the time. Now nobody even walks to school. I just think people need to walk more, and it would be great if our cities were designed so that we could walk to places, because it seems like walking is a chore. We're such a car-dependent society. Just walk more throughout the day.

#7: Stand up more. People just sit so much. Even if you're in your office, try to stand for five minutes every hour instead of sitting behind the desk. Try to keep your core strong, because as we age, everybody just starts having all these back problems. We sit too much, and we don't walk enough.

#8: Sometimes, less really IS more. My thing is to educate people and get them to realize they don't need to spend hours upon hours on a treadmill to get the results they want.

#9: Muscle is where it's at. I think it's important for women to realize that as we age, we lose muscle mass unless we do something to prevent that loss, and that's what generally causes middle-age weight gain. You're not really doing anything different, but all of a sudden, your clothes don't fit right and your stomach's bigger; it's because you're losing muscles. That's also what is contributing to bone loss and osteoporosis. So, I just think women need to know it's really important to do some sort of strength resistance training as they age to not only keep their weight down, but to prevent bone loss.

#10: Not all food is created equal. I think people need to realize they have to eat good food. Half the battle is the exercise, but you've got to pay attention to what you're putting in your mouth, too.

#11: Eat five times a day. I try to get my clients to eat five times a day: breakfast, snack, lunch, snack, and dinner. I try to get them to eat all real food. So, a 100-calorie snack pack would not be something I would recommend. You're trying to get the most nutritional bang for your calorie buck, so eat real whole foods like fruit, yogurt, and nuts.

#12: Fruits are fine, but veggies are divine. I always challenge people to eat more vegetables, because I think it's easy to add more fruit to your diet, but I think it's a lot harder to get the veggies in. So, I always challenge people to eat as much green food as they can.

So there you have it, a dozen great excuse-dumping habits to live by from a great personal trainer who learned the hard way that life doesn't have to get in the way of feeling and looking your best!

Chapter 3

Finding Your Passion
with **Ashley Borden**

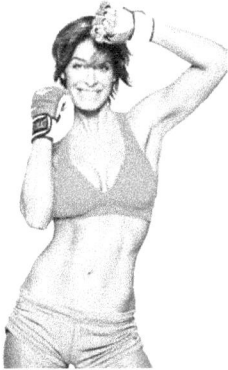

"Learning something new is really great for your body. Learn new movement patterns you haven't done, like taking dance class or salsa night every Thursday, or learning a new sport."
~ Ashley Borden

Ashley Borden is a fitness and lifestyle consultant to some of Hollywood's most recognizable faces and world-class athletes.

Her unique approach to fitness can be attributed to tackling her own personal struggles and transforming them into a positive philosophy and a dynamic training program, making her one of the most sought-after experts in her field.

Her humor-laced candor suits all types of high-profile clients, including Christina Aguilera, Natasha Bedingfield, Mandy Moore, and Ryan Gosling, as well as Nick Swisher of the New

York Yankees and UFC champion Matt Hughes. Borden also works as a master trainer with fellow trainers and coaches.

Borden's tips and techniques have been featured in *InStyle*, *Vogue*, *Elle*, *Allure*, *Departures*, and the *Los Angeles Times*, to name a few. Most recently, she can be seen on The Cooking Channel's new show *Drop 5 Lbs*. as a cohost. She is also an advisor for Livestrong.com and *Fitness* magazine.

Women's Health named Borden a top Body Transformer in 2011, one of only six trainers in the country. Internationally, she has been recognized by publications such as *Elle Japan*, *Harper's Bazaar* Russia, *Who* Australia and London's *NOW* magazine. In addition, she has been a featured expert on the Today Show, Rachael Ray, Discovery Health, the Tyra Banks Show, MTV, VH1, E! Entertainment, and more.

Publisher McGraw-Hill debuted her book *Your Perfect Fit*, which she coauthored with denim designer Paige Adams-Geller (of Paige Denim) in 2008. The book, the first to marry fashion, fitness, and Borden's SOS food plan, was given kudos by the *Wall Street Journal*. She has also released two training DVDs with the global health media company Gaiam, and was the technical fitness director for UFC star Matt Hughes's fitness DVD.

After a successful three-year run at the Four Seasons Punta Mita, Mexico, Borden brought her private and corporate luxury fitness retreats to the 5-star Pelican Hill Resort in Newport Beach, California. The four-day experience included personal training, spa treatments, and customized meals by the executive chef according to Borden's SOS food plan. Her retreats are now available to be tailored for individuals or companies at any resort property.

Borden volunteers with the physical rehabilitation of breast cancer survivors, and through the Chaka Khan Foundation, she has helped at-risk youth and children improve their knowledge of nutrition and fitness.

An avid dancer growing up, she always felt an inherent connection to fitness, yet battled a vicious eating disorder throughout her teen years. Hitting bottom at age eighteen, Borden finally found a peaceful balance between exercise and nutrition through Overeaters Anonymous. "After having such a profound recovery experience, I felt inspired to share my insight on exercise and nutrition with others," she says.

Originally from Chicago, Ashley has been living and working in the training and fitness fields full-time for over two decades. Borden currently trains privately at Fitness Factory in Los Angeles. Ashley recalls her rocky road into the fitness and nutrition industry: "My mom owned a health food store for eleven years. It was a big part of my upbringing, but it was never explained to me why I couldn't have sugar or any of this other stuff. The whole issue of food not being allowed kind of triggered a want for something because I wasn't allowed to have it when I was younger, so I developed an eating disorder when I was in fourth grade, and I hit bottom when I was seventeen. I went to a treatment center. I was anorexic, bulimic, a compulsive overeater, and a compulsive exerciser. My recovery was finding a balance between training and food."

Ashley knew she had to come to terms with her excessive thoughts and feelings about food, exercise, and living a balanced life. "So when I got out of treatment, that's when I decided: I love training, but it had been such a nightmare for me and for my health, meaning, my own working out. I wanted to find a balance, but I didn't know how to live a lean, livable lifestyle and not feel ill. So that's what my goal was for my own recovery, but my training was also what drove me."

Arriving in Los Angeles was a fresh start in more ways than one, as Ashley recalls. "When I started training in Los Angeles, I only trained women because that's what resonated with me the most in the beginning. That was really my main passion that got me started, and I really needed to help other people find the balance that I had finally found after so my many years of suffering. That was my mission, and still is to this day, and then everything else totally fell into place business-wise. When I was in high school, I didn't know I wanted to be a trainer, or I would have gone to college for it. I didn't even know that was an option. I had no idea."

What's great about Ashley, not just as a professional but as a trainer, is the empathy she brings to both roles. "My own recovery is what's helped me connect so well with people," she says, "and I have the ability to explain things in a way that people understand. I don't like it when people explain science or fitness to me in a patronizing way. I try to be the liaison between the information and the clients by making it accessible for them."

When it comes to personal training, Ashley uses a three-part approach. "I go through a full body assessment of all their biomechanics and movement patterns, and then we go through full body warm-up. After warm-up, then it's into conditioning focus. The focus of my training is to bring everybody as close to their anatomically correct position as possible. So the focus is on posture. Basically everybody nowadays has a weak posterior chain because they all sit at a computer all day long."

Naturally, someone with as much expertise as Ashley is going to have some advice for readers about how to overcome excuses, resistance, and intimidation to create your more healthy, happy, and fit YOU in twelve secrets or less. So, here in a nutshell are Ashley's "dirty dozen" fitness, nutrition, and health tips.

Top 12 Tips from Ashley

#1: Plan to succeed. When most people don't have a sustainable workout system, it's because they're not pre-planning; they're just flying by the seat of their pants with their schedule. I schedule for my whole life, every week before. It's my appointments. I have it in front of me on my computer. My workouts are preplanned, my time is preplanned, because otherwise I won't do it.

#2: See the bigger picture. You need to first work backward and ask yourself, "So, what is the issue? What is the block?"

It could be a mom saying, "I have no time in the morning."

My response is, "Okay, well why not?"

She says, "Because I'm getting my kids ready."

I ask, "Okay, but what about getting up earlier?" "I can't."

"Why not?"

"I'm exhausted."

"Why?"

"Because I go to bed so late."

"Why?"

"Because I don't get anything done during the day."

"Why?"

"Because I don't have it planned, and I'm just running around like a chicken with my head cut off all day long, and I don't even have it written down."

"Oh, okay. So, let's start there."

So it's a domino effect of discovering where the problem is. You have to play detective with your life and say, "Okay, what in the world is going on?" Look at all your excuses, keep on backing up and asking yourself why, and you'll usually find where the issue is.

#3: Don't do everything; do *something*. You can't play the all-or-nothing game with training and with your food. I always tell people that it's not about being perfect and doing everything. It's about doing something. So, when I go on vacation, I always train in the morning. I get up, make sure I have my coffee, and then I train. Whether that training is power walking on the beach or inside the gym—whatever it is, I break a sweat and do some sort of exercise. And I have one hour where I roll out with my body—I warm up and do those exercises. Then I can get into the rest of the day, and I'm totally relaxed. But I also don't go on vacation and suddenly start eating every single horrible food that I'd never eat in my life. I'll still eat dark chocolate, but it'll be dark chocolate that doesn't have partially hydrogenated fats in it. I tell people, "You go on vacation, but your body doesn't want to vacation." And it's not an all-or-nothing thing. It's that mentality of thinking, *Oh, I'm on vacation; I am not going to take care of myself.* That's more abusive than it is a vacation. Then you come back and wonder what the heck you did! So okay, so if you're not training every day, that's fine, so then do this: make sure you're pounding your water, and maybe you brought your baby roller with you and roll out every day, or you're going to do a walk every day for an hour. You do some kind of negotiation with yourself so that it's not all or nothing.

#4: Layer your goals. You have to be realistic. It's a LIFESTYLE change, so it doesn't happen overnight.

#5: Stay positive. I always tell people, "I want you to write down the positive things you see." You always remember the negative stuff; you never remember the good. Maybe you write something like, "I ate like crap there." You don't write down, "I drank all my water today, and I didn't eat any crappy food, and I even trained for half an hour!" Write down one positive thing every day that you've done toward changing your lifestyle. Keep these in a little notebook so that you can see all your positives.

#6: Don't go it alone. I got to the point where I could not get excited about training myself by myself anymore. I tried joining a nice gym. I couldn't stand it. I don't want to be in a gym any more than necessary because I'm in a gym all day long, so I hired Brian, my trainer. I train with him three days a week.

#7: Try something new. Learning something new is really great for your body. Learn new movement patterns you haven't done before, like taking dance class or salsa night every Thursday, or learning a new sport. Go outside your comfort box or your comfort zone. This will also challenge your body physically because you will be doing something you've never done.

#8: Choose your environment carefully. My stepdad is a senior (competence) attorney for the seventh appellate court, so he sits all day long. He is the smartest man in the entire world, but he was getting a little older, and he was not training. I could see it in his body; it was like his body was kind of falling apart a little bit, and it was making me really upset. My mom is a machine—she's a training animal. My mom is in the best shape of her life, and she is sixty-seven years old. And so the problem with my dad was that he didn't know how to train. So he really did need to have a trainer, and it had to be in an environment where he felt safe and comfortable, which was his home. So my mom got him a trainer for ten sessions, and he started loving it because he was learning in an environment where he didn't feel intimidated, and his trainer is a very good instructor. Now that he's training, he feels good about himself, and he's making much better choices with his food That makes me so happy because I want to see him get strong.

#9: Don't be intimidated. My dad has always loved to hike, but I don't think he truly understood what it meant to feel strong yet, because he had never really done it. So it wasn't his forte. I think he felt a little intimidated by it. Because my mom was a dancer, exercising was very natural for her, but it wasn't as natural for my stepdad.

#10: Dig deeper. One of my favorite quotes is that, "Just because a gym is public doesn't mean you're supposed to know how to use it." If you have a bad experience, it's traumatizing. And why would you ever want to go back? You know what I mean? I usually like to figure out what my clients are asking; what are the real reasons they're at the gym? It's a very good thing to find out why. What is it about the exercise that they don't like?

#11: Hydrate yourself. When your body is hydrated, you don't crave food as much. Your skin is much more supple, and you actually look better, because it's more plump and filled up. Hydration decreases headaches and helps you focus. I think probably ninety percent of people are dehydrated. Most people don't drink enough water at all.

#12: Lose the soda: Never drink another soda as long as you live. My mom used to drink Diet Coke. She drank about four cans of it a day. She was very addicted to Diet Coke, too. She dropped the Diet Coke and lost eight pounds. All that soda does is bloat you. Your body is made up of zero percent Diet Coke. Ok, I mean, you have no Diet Coke in your body at all, and you are drinking nothing but chemicals. You are drinking one hundred percent fizzy chemicals that bloat you. So you might not even know that you're bloated, but when you stop drinking soda, that you will lose the bloat, especially in your stomach. There is no reason on earth to drink soda.

I want to thank Ashley for making such great contributions to this book. She really has a lot to say, as all these trainers do, and I found her 12 secrets to be especially helpful. I hope you did as well. If you want to know more about Ashley, or would like instructions on "rolling out," visit her at www.ashleyborden.com.

Chapter 4

Getting Personal
with **David Vaughan**

*"Physiologically, the only thing that's ever been proven to reduce your weight is to **eat less** and **do more**."*
~ David Vaughan

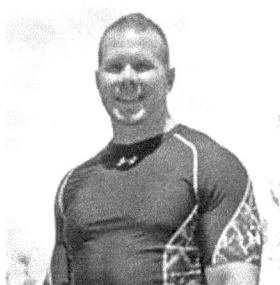

Personal trainer David Vaughan is committed to helping his clients improve their quality of life by sharing the knowledge and experience that he has gained during his fourteen-year career in health, fitness, and athletic conditioning. David prides himself on professionalism, courtesy, and constantly studying and striving to be the best trainer he can be.

He has helped hundreds of clients reach their specific fitness and athletic goals. These clients have ranged in age from seven to ninety-nine, and have included high school athletes, collegiate athletes, professional athletes, amateur and professional golfers, work-at-home moms, a former Mrs. Illinois pageant winner, aspiring bodybuilders, patients with Alzheimer's

disease, Cystic Fibrosis, and Parkinson's disease, cardiac rehabilitation patients, and physical therapy patients. These clients
have all needed specific programs to gain specific results.

Since moving to Las Vegas in 2005 David has worked with
several local professional athletes, entrepreneurs, poker pros,
news personalities, entertainers such as Barry Manilow, and the
cast of *The Phantom of the Opera*.

Like many young kids, David was introduced to fitness
through sports. He recalls, "I was always playing a lot of sports
when I was a teenager, and working out and weightlifting was
the baseline for football. I had a hockey coach who wanted us
to work out and weight-lift, so I was always doing something
along those lines. And even after I quit athletics, I continued
working out, and then I went to college with the idea of, *Hey,
I'll be a physical therapist.*"

Eventually, David's interests shifted from the more technical
aspect of his career choice to the physical. He explains, "What
I liked most was taking the holistic approach to helping people
recondition their bodies. I was really drawn to injury preven-
tion, particularly the post-rehab portion of it versus the weight
loss and transformation aspect of it.

"As I studied, my training and conscience evolved. I really
loved the fact that I could be creative once I learned the basic
planes of the body as well as the basic movements and pos-
tures. I could be very creative with what I did, and then I could
come up with something different every day to challenge my
clients and myself."

Now that he trains clients full-time, David has found a passion for inspiring them as well. "I'm always looking for something different for my clients to keep workouts interesting;
that's why they hire a trainer," he explains. "I mean, if you want
to train you could just go to the gym, get on a treadmill, ride

a bike, or go around and do all ten machines that are there, or whatever, so your job is to basically just inspire people."

David is proud of his career, as well as his gym. When asked about his mission statement, David explains, "The mission of Forget the Gym is to provide safe, high-quality fitness training for the residents of the Las Vegas Valley. In doing so, we support all of our clients in their efforts to reach their fitness goals. Forget The Gym provides professional fitness trainers to people of all ages and abilities. We provide industry-leading health and wellness professionals to ensure clients get the results they deserve. Forget the Gym is committed to providing support and encouragement to the clients we serve."

David likes to keep his trainers on their toes and is diligent about providing the finest quality service for his clients. He adds, "We actually have eight personal trainers who work for us, and so we have monthly continuing education seminars, just within our own little group, because all trainers are required to have a national certification.

"But in my experience through the years, trainers get lazy over time, and they kind of adopt one style, and that's what they want to do: they want to be a bodybuilder, they want to be a sports trainer, they want to do this or that."

Considering he's based in Las Vegas, it should come as no surprise that some of David's best clients spend most of their days inside a casino. "I train a lot of professional poker players in their younger twenties," he explains. "And they all want to be trained as if they are professional athletes, which is kind of funny considering the sport—if you want to call it that, but they're competitive. So they kind of have that athletic mindset a little bit, and maybe that translates into training.

"They're doing forty-yard sprints, and it's five thousand dollars to whoever wins the best of five, so it gets really interesting.

And they always have weight loss bets; for instance, one of my current clients only signed up because he needs to lose weight before the World Series, and he gets something like ten thousand dollars for every one percent of weight he loses."

David also enjoys a fair amount of clients from the other end of the competitive and age spectrum. As he says, "I personally have a fifty-fifty mix between older people and poker players. The older clients are generally working to lower their blood pressure, lower their cholesterol levels, and attain overall health and longevity. They're just trying to look better and feel better. And then I have the other end of the spectrum, which is the poker players, but there's not a whole lot in between. And so I've got sixty- and seventy-year-olds in a room next to twenty- and thirty-year-old poker players. But I can go from taking someone for a power walk for fifteen to twenty minutes in the morning and working on balance stuff, to by the afternoon we're doing kickboxing, Muay Thai, or sprinting down the field, and they're towing me!"

David is particularly excited about a new offering that he is using with his clients called a BOD POD. He explains, "It's basically the gold standard in body fat testing. Everybody always uses calipers or the bioelectrical scales, and there's so much error involved in those that I just thought, *Hey, you know what? I'm sick of telling my clients, 'Well, it could be this or it could be that,'* so I obtained a BOD POD. It measures air displacement. You sit inside it, and the whole test actually takes two minutes as it measures temperature, air pressure, and air displacement."

Although he works with twelve to fourteen clients per week, David likes to put the personal in personal training. "You shouldn't have a blueprint for everyone," he believes. "You should sit down with the person, assess what their goals are, assess what their weaknesses are, determine what they can and can't do, and define it from there. Each person is different as far as what's going to keep them motivated and having fun, so you've got to tailor the program to the person."

David has some pretty strong thoughts on nutritional supplements. "I don't recommend a whole lot of nutritional supplements," he explains, "because I was taught in college that ninety-nine percent of them are BS because of the way the supplement industry is. Nothing's really regulated. All they have to prove is that it doesn't harm you; it doesn't actually have to be proven to work. So I only recommend multivitamins or proteins. If it doesn't hurt my clients, I allow them to buy it."

David likes to meet with his clients, on average, he says, "Three days. There are people I see every day, but if I had to average it, I'd say three. I always recommend three days for people because you want them to do some workouts on their own."

David stresses the importance of both short- and long-term goals, and he explains the difference. "A long-term goal might be, 'Shear my body fat down to six or seven percent,' and a short-term goal might be, 'I'm going on vacation in six weeks, and I want to look really good in the photos.'"

David insists that going on vacation can be a good thing for your exercise regimen, and that most of his clients benefit from the experience. "When people go on vacation, my whole goal is for them to try to stay the same weight as they were when they left. I don't want them to gain anything; I don't expect them to lose anything."

Now that we've gotten to know him a little better, it's time for David to share some specifics on how to get and stay healthy. So here are David's top 12 tips on how to get and keep your *more healthy, happy, and fit YOU.*

Top 12 Tips from David

#1: Make lifestyle choices that are easy to maintain. People set these very aggressive goals, and then they get really frustrated when they only lose three pounds within a week or something like that. They eat only salads, and they follow a totally non-maintainable diet for two or three weeks, and they'll lose a ridiculous number of pounds, anywhere from fifteen to twenty pounds, but it's just not going to be maintainable. And then, what ends up happening is they think, *Oh, that was so easy*, and they usually go out and gorge for a few days. And then they don't get back to their diet right away, and the next thing you know, they're actually a few pounds heavier than when they started. On their own, these are just people that I know that have gone and have stepped off on programs and got a little too gung-ho from the start, instead of trying to make the lifestyle changes.

#2: It's okay to take a break—just not indefinitely. A lot of people who work out pretty regularly eventually realize that they should take a week off every so often and let their central nervous system relax. And so those people who have usually worked out about a year straight, who never really took some time off and just stayed on their regimen might say, 'Oh, I'm going to take off this week.' They do that, but during the next go-round, it creeps into a week and a half, and then every break takes a little longer to the point where eventually you might not work out at all anymore.

#3: Avoid stress eating. Over the years when working with clients, I've seen many people become stress eaters. I think it's just a comfort thing.

#4: Eat less, do more—period. Physiologically, the only thing that's ever been proven to reduce your weight is <u>eat less</u> and <u>do more</u>.

#5: Choose your food wisely. People need to become a little more educated on food choices; just pay more attention to reading food labels. A really cheap, easy way to become fit is to look at the labels of the foods you're eating. Look at the nutritional information on the label. Realize when you go to McDonald's and order a breaded chicken sandwich that it's not the same as a grilled chicken sandwich.

#6: Watch your sodium. Definitely look at the sodium content in whatever you're eating. If it's pre-packaged, the sodium content is always going to be high. I don't know why people have trouble understanding that sodium is a good preservative in a lot of things. You want to eat fresh foods anyway. You can find fresh foods if you shop the perimeter of the grocery store.

#7: Count ALL your calories. Always look at total calories versus serving size, because a lot of foods are labeled *only 200 calories*, but that is per serving, and then you realize that the serving is two ounces, but you ate the whole thing! And then you want to look at fat grams, and how much sugar is in the food, and those are all actually in bold print on the label, so you don't have to look too far to find them.

#8: Finding the right fit with your trainer is key. You want somebody who is living the lifestyle without overindulging in it. When someone keeps talking about his or her accomplishments—that's somebody who's not for you, 'cause they're a little too into themselves.

#9: Find a trainer that appreciates flexibility. You want someone who listens to you and makes adjustments. There's going to be a point where you need to be pushed, but there's also a point where something may physically hurt you.

#10: Find a trainer who listens. Something may be going on in your personal life, and you want someone who's going to listen to you and know how to handle that situation with you. You want someone who will be flexible, and at the same time, be strong.

#11: Be in it to win it. For the most part, I tell my clients, "It's the home stretch—last ten minutes," because people are usually dead tired by the end of the workout, and I just want to keep them going, so I encourage them that they're in the homestretch, near the end.

#12: Don't underestimate the power of fun! We're all about having fun. Everyone's kind of on the same page. We have a little meeting with our clients in the beginning and get a feel for what their personalities are, and ninety percent of the clients enjoy humor. We get them moving and keep them moving. For the ones who are really intense about working out, all we have to say is, "Let's go!"

Great tips, David! But then, I'd expect nothing less from a guy who is so committed, passionate, and focused on helping everyone he comes in contact with find their own better body—on their own terms!

Chapter 5

Give Yourself 10 Minutes
with **Franklin Antoian**

"Just ease into it; just try ten minutes; that's a good key number. Even if it's just ten minutes, it's one hundred percent more than what you were doing before."
~ Franklin Antoian

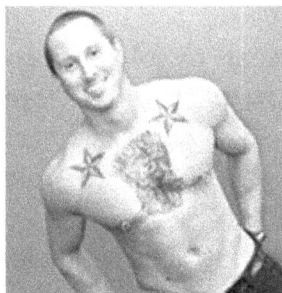

ACE certified personal trainer and fitness expert Franklin Antoian is so committed to his clients, he is available to them 24/7: online!

The owner and founder of iBodyFit.com, Franklin helps clients reach peak levels of physical fitness through both in-home and online personal training sessions. "I genuinely love getting people fit and healthy," he says.

This passion not only prompted Franklin to become a personal trainer, but to found his website and pen two books, *The Fit Executive* and *Top Ten Ab Exercises*, as well as additional articles on health and wellness.

Personal training isn't the only way Franklin spreads his knowledge of health and wellness, either. He also schools clients on basic nutrition know-how, as he believes the two go hand in hand. From what snacks to eat to what vitamins need supplementing, Franklin has a wealth of knowledge on nutrition and health, and is ready and willing to share.

Former and current clients aren't shy about testifying to the amazing results they've achieved on Franklin's watch. Besides taking the guess-work out of exercise, he also motivates clients who are convinced they will never lose weight or get in shape to believe that anything and everything is possible.

How does he keep going day after day?

Franklin says it's simple. "I do what I love."

Unlike a lot of professionals in the fitness field, Franklin started in another industry altogether. "I've always worked out and liked fitness, but I actually had a different career before this. I was in the financial field. I lived in New York and worked at the Stock Exchange, doing that crazy yelling and screaming stuff. But after doing that for five or six years or so, I decided to kind of do what I want to do. I heard this quote, 'If you love what you do, you'll never have to work again.' So I said, 'Let me just try to make a living with this and try and help people get fit.'"

Franklin's approach to his own fitness goals is fairly simple. "My exercise program is kind of basic," he explains. "For me, the basics are whatever gets you fit. In other words, there's a certain amount of time for me that you're supposed to do your cardio training, your strength training, and flexibility training. And I stick to those guidelines along with a great nutrition plan, and that works for me."

Franklin's recommendations for others wanting a varied but effective fitness regimen are equally basic: "For cardio training, it's five days a week for a minimum of thirty minutes. For strength training, it's a minimum of two times a week for about thirty minutes. And stretching is just pretty much every day."

When it comes to obtaining a better body, Franklin's philosophy is all-inclusive. "Fitness is for everybody," he says, "not just for a certain amount of people. It's for anybody, not just for someone who's trying to lose weight, but for whoever. You can gain effectively at muscle and strengthen your heart up at any age, whether old or young."

Speaking of ages, Franklin's average client is thirty to fifty years old, has a family, and has a full-time job. They come to see him early in the morning or early in the evening, before or after their crazy heavy days, and yet they still work out. Then again, there are always exceptions.

"My youngest client is twenty-four," he adds. "My oldest one is ninety-four!"

Franklin works with about fifteen to twenty different people each week in his gym, but he also makes it affordable to get hands-on advice and input from a personal trainer through his iBodyFit.com program where, for less than a hundred dollars, you can get a month of professional training online.

Why do we often fall off the wagon on our path to a better body? Franklin has some specific thoughts about why people stop and start their weight loss, fitness, and nutrition goals. "I think a lot of people fall off that wagon because they just go at it too hard," he explains.

As always, Franklin makes such good points! Now I want to collect them all here in Franklin's top 12 recommendations for obtaining your own better body—on your own terms.

Top 12 Tips from Franklin

#1: Get a workout program that fits you. You don't want to try to do too much, especially in the beginning. People who tend to do that get burned out, and then they just fall apart; they get unmotivated, they get injured, they get tired, and then they just don't want to go back.

#2: Mix it up every three months. If you just mix up your routine to get rid of any type of boredom, that's probably a good thing. Boredom is one of the top reasons that people fall out of their routines.

#3: Take a vacation from exercise. Give your body a break. When you come back, get a new routine and try that after a few months, and then at the end of another three months try another routine, so let's go with boredom as an answer for that.

#4: Avoid doing too much too soon. People just go out, they haven't worked out or done anything in forever or a long time, and they'll just try to go to the gym every day. They'll try to lift weights that are too heavy for them, they'll try to run too far too long, and they'll either get discouraged because they can't do what they thought they could, or they won't fit, or they get injured because the weights they're lifting are too heavy.

#5: Don't set such huge goals for yourself right away. Don't say, "I need to lose fifty pounds." Just set a small goal: "I gotta lose ten pounds, and I gotta lose it by two months from now." Then, after two months, reassess and go from there.

#6: Give yourself ten minutes. Just ease into it; just try ten minutes; that's a good key number. Even if it's just ten minutes, it's one hundred percent more than what you were doing before. You'll be so surprised if you do a quick weight workout for ten minutes, especially if you've done nothing in a year. But the difference you'll feel is that your muscles will get stronger, and mentally you'll feel great, because you've just worked out. Soon, you'll find yourself doing ten, fifteen, twenty minutes; the next thing you know, you're working out an hour.

#7: Avoid the world's top three excuses for not working out! What most people say about not exercising is that they don't have enough time to work out. (And that's probably because of the myth about how long a workout takes.) So, they think they don't have enough time, they don't know what to do, and a lot of people say, "I don't like gyms."

#8: Exercise can be fun. Ignore the misinformation or lack of information about working out. A lot of people think that in order to do a cardio workout, for example, you have to be sweaty, out of breath, running, and pushing, pushing, pushing yourself. And the truth is, it's finding a workout you can live with. Just do something that elevates your heart rate, from running to playing Frisbee to chasing your kids around the park, to biking; it can be something fun.

#9: You don't have to walk much, but walk every day. You should walk for thirty minutes every day. It's going to lower your chances of heart disease.

#10: Show some resistance. Do some kind of resistance or strength training, such as push-ups, sit-ups, or just basic stuff that you can do for free. You can do simple things in the park or at home—very, very simple training exercises that will make your posture better and increase your stamina and strength.

#11: Stretch for your health. I recommend quite a bit of stretching. If you do just these things to increase your lifespan, you will see an improvement in lifestyle.

#12: Control what you can control. You are the only person in control of your body—not your boss, not your kid, not your spouse, not your mom, not anybody. You're the only one who is going to make yourself work out, eat healthy, and change your body. Your boss can tell you go to work, your spouse can yell at you, your kids can choose not to listen to you; you don't have control over that stuff, really. But you do have control over your body and what you do to it, and what you put in it— that's what I'm trying to say. No matter what is going on, one thing that you have control over is your body.

This is all such good advice, and I have a feeling Franklin could go on all day like this! I encourage you to visit iBodyFit.com to learn more about Franklin and discover for yourself how he helps people go from "wannabes" to "yeah, baby!"

Chapter 6

Get Your Body in Motion
with **Gilad Janklowicz**

*"Never completely exhaust yourself because of the workout.
Always walk away from a workout with something left."*
*~ **Gilad Janklowicz***

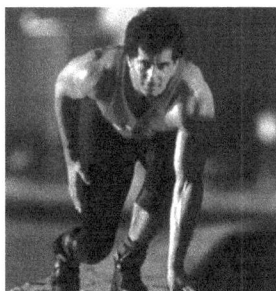

Gilad Janklowicz is one of the world's most popular fitness personalities. As a pioneer in the fitness industry, he has helped millions to stay fit with his popular TV fitness shows *Bodies in Motion*, *Basic Training the Workout* and *Total Body Sculpt with Gilad* and with his gold and platinum instructional home fitness DVDs and videos.

Filmed on location in the beautiful Hawaiian Islands, *Bodies in Motion* is a half-hour aerobic and toning workout show that launched in 1983. It was the first fitness show to air on ESPN, where it enjoyed an eleven-year run from 1985 to 1996.

From 1996 to 2002, the show aired on Fox Sports and on The Health Network. As of 2002, the show has been airing on

Discovery's new fitness channel FitTV. Currently, the show is the longest-running fitness show in the United States.

Bodies in Motion aired in over eighty countries and was chosen as the number one TV fitness program in the world by *Self* magazine. In a viewers' poll conducted by FitTV, Gilad won the title of Fitness Instructor of the Year for the years 2004, 2005, 2006, and 2007.

In January 2005, Gilad released *Total Body Sculpt with Gilad*. This series was created for FitTV to complement the existing *Bodies in Motion* show and give the viewers a dynamic new concept in fitness that focuses on sculpting exercises and strength training. Forty shows have been taped to date.

Gilad also created an exercise program for ESPN entitled *Basic Training the Workout*, a boot camp style training program hosted by his sister, Ada. The program debuted in 1988 and aired for five years.

Most of Gilad's life has been devoted to fitness since high school where he excelled in track and field. He eventually became a record-holding decathlon athlete in Israel and a fitness officer in the military. Later, as an Olympic hopeful in 1980, he trained and competed alongside some of the best athletes in the world. Gilad was inducted into the Jewish Sports Hall of Fame in 1991.

After an Achilles injury shattered his Olympic dreams, Gilad enrolled at the UCLA film school and began instructing fitness classes in some of Los Angeles's top studios and fitness facilities where he built a strong following and trained some of the world's best-known celebrities.

Fitness personalities such as Arnold Schwarzenegger, Jack LaLanne, and quarterback Joe Theismann all trained with Gilad and appeared on his television program *Bodies in Motion*.

You know Gilad.

Or, if you don't, you know *of* him. You've probably seen his face, as well as his fit body, staring back at you from the television screen as you've flipped through the channels.

Despite hosting two television shows and filming videos all year long, Gilad still finds time to teach classes during his hectic and busy travel schedule.

"I do teach off and on," he explains, "in town or in different places across the country when I'm traveling. A lot of the work that we do is geared toward our production, which is new videos, new DVDs, and new shows."

Gilad finds that teaching between big productions helps inform his newer projects. "I get ideas from talking to people, working with people, and seeing what motivates them, what doesn't motivate them, and what they're looking for in a fitness program. And then, I also make sure that I'm pretty much updated; I speak to new trends, although I don't always follow the trends. But I take new, innovative things in fitness, and I try to incorporate them into my own style as well. I've been doing this for years, and I try to keep everything very, very simple for the viewer."

Unlike many of the trainers we spoke with who were strictly hands-on, Gilad is unique in that his television show reaches so many viewers. "When you reach the audience through television," Gilad explains, "it's a complicated thing because there's a variety of audience members. You have people who are really fit, all the way to people who are completely out of shape and overweight.

"I don't really know who I'm reaching out there. I just know that I'm reaching people, but I try to make it in such a way that everybody gets something out of it. In other words, if I have someone who's a complete beginner, who's never worked out before, and has forty to fifty pounds to lose, and he's at home, there's something on the show for him. It's not going to be too hard for him that he can't do it, and the moves are not going to be so complicated that he can't follow.

"If I have somebody who's more advanced, who wants to use the show as a good overall workout, it will invite him to do that. In other words, it doesn't gear to the beginners or to the advanced. It kinda gives it the middle of the road."

What kind of training does Gilad do to stay fit? "I do a variety of things," he says in response. "I teach a variety of classes, so that helps me stay in shape. I do some strength training and toning sometimes at the gym, sometimes outdoors. I walk and hike every so often. I do some swimming. And when I'm gearing up to do our production, I kinda increase the intensity a little bit so I can get into really tip-top shape."

Most of the trainers I spoke with looked up to at least someone in their industry, and Gilad is no exception, but he has had several mentors, not just one.

"I've had a couple of mentors over the years," he adds. "One of them was, of course, the legendary Jack LaLanne. I've also had another mentor who was a little bit older than Jack LaLanne, and actually lived a little longer, too.

"But he wasn't necessarily anyone that anybody would know. His name was Erwin Jaskulski, and he was a very fit man who broke some Guinness world record, and lived here in Hawaii, and we were very good friends for many, many years.

"He was a close friend and a mentor, and actually very inspiring.

He passed away in 2006 at the age of one hundred three and a half, competing all the way 'til he was one hundred two. He actually established and broke all these world records in the track and field events: one hundred meters, two hundred meters, and four hundred- meter dashes. It goes by five-year increments.

"When he turned ninety, he broke a couple of world records. When he turned ninety-five, he broke two and established one, and when he turned one hundred, he broke and established three world records."

When asked about his mentors outside of the fitness arena, Gilad has a surprising answer—or perhaps not so surprising when you hear why. "I'm a big admirer of Clint Eastwood," he explains, "because it's amazing the amount of stuff he does, and given his age that he's able to keep getting better. And I think as he goes along and produces or directs films or acts in them, I think he just keeps getting better.

"That's very inspiring, because a lot of people reach a certain age and retire. It's just amazing to see someone who has had so much success along his life, just keep getting better at it. I actually got to meet him in person and got an autograph, which I was very excited about."

Thanks to the popularity of his long-running television series and video workouts, Gilad has a wide target audience. "I don't see a specific gender in mind," he explains. "I don't see a specific condition in mind. What I see is someone at home who's looking for inspiration. I'm trying to think, *What does that person look for, and what does he want to hear from me, and what does he want to see me do?*

"That's what I keep my mind on. So if I'm talking through the show, if I'm saying things, or if I'm just kinda joking around, whatever it is, I'm trying to get to the point that I'm pulling that viewer with me into the workout, and working out with them hand in hand.

"So that's my whole idea. Rather than do fancy footsteps to show them what I can do, I try to go, 'Listen, hey, you can do this, too. Get off your couch. Follow what I'm doing. I'll take you through it' and that's my motto."

As one might imagine, Gilad has met with a wide range of adoring and faithful fans over the years. "We've had some amazing responses from people," he begins. "I've had professional boxers who see me on the street go, 'Wow, I've been working out to your show.' I had a few stars say, 'Wow, you're Gilad. Hey, I've been watching you for years.' I've had some overweight housewives, and ladies who just gave birth—all kinds. I've had people say, 'I moved to Hawaii because of you, because I saw your show in London.' I mean, I've had the whole gamut."

What does Gilad think about his fans' reactions? "It legitimizes what I'm doing," he says, "and it tells me I'm on the right track as far as the way I think about going about it. And sometimes it's almost embarrassing, because the responses are so good that I'm thinking, *Wow, this is really working.* It's very rewarding.

"We just had a fitness camp on the Big Island here, our third one that we do every year. We have people come here from all over the world. We were about forty in total. We did a week-long fitness camp, and it's amazing 'cause you really see how you touched their lives with this TV show. They're saying things that, seriously—I'm sitting there and I'm feeling embarrassed in a way, but it's very complimentary, and it's amazing to see the kind of effect you have through this medium."

Every fitness expert has a preferred way of working out and working with clients. Gilad is no different, and here he offers his main priorities with any workout. "First of all, one of the most important things for me is body placement, posture, and making sure that I always go from the light to the more advanced.

"I used to run track and field, and one of the things I learned very early on is that no matter what workout you do, you always need to do a good warmup and a good stretch to prepare the body for more intense moves.

"So with every one of my workouts I'm always very adamant about giving a very good warm-up, then of course focusing on the three most important elements of fitness, which are cardiovascular endurance, strength training and toning, and stretching and flexibility."

For peak conditioning, Gilad recommends doing at least something physical every day. "It has to be a variety of different things," he adds. "Let's say, for example, on a Monday you would be focusing more on cardiovascular fitness. Tuesday you would be focusing a little bit more on sculpting and toning. Wednesday you would focus on core and stretching. There's a variety of ways to do this, but, in general, you need a lot of variety in the workout, not the same thing day after day."

Since his televised workouts are what helped make Gilad such an instantly recognized international fitness expert and worldwide TV star, it should come as no surprise that his specially designed DVDs are still incredibly popular.

He explains, "We have individual videos. You can build up a library with them. And you have anything from abdominal specific workouts, to step workouts, to kickboxing workouts, to sculpting workouts, to toning workouts at advanced, intermediate—different levels.

"On the DVDs," he continues, "we have some that are specifically created systems. We have what we call the Ultimate Body Sculpt, which is actually a three-pack of videos, and it kind of targets different muscle groups and different functions of fitness in each one of the DVDs.

"We have one that's called the Quick Fit System, which is a series of seven workouts. It comes with a diet plan, an exercise guide, a journal, and a CD to explain it—and that's a system all on its own. And then we have the newest one we did, which is called Lord of the Abs.

"It's a five-pack; five different workouts. The average time is about fifty minutes per workout, and it basically targets everything that's got to do with your core, but it's not just sit-ups. It's standing core workout with a heavy ball. It's sole workout with a heavy ball. It's cardio moves like martial arts and boxing and kickboxing style moves, all issues related to the core. We have a circuit interval training that involves cardio and core, as well as the upper body."

As if that's not enough to crow about, Gilad is particularly excited about his series of short workout programs called the Express Workouts, which include fifteen workouts on two DVDs, all under ten minutes each.

Gilad explains, "So somebody who's at work and just wants to have a quick break and a ten-minute workout, and then get back to the desk, awesome. Wake up in the morning, you want to do a ten-minute workout before you go to work, get your body moving, awesome. It does have everything."

Gilad adds, "So we have a variety of different things to offer people different styles of workouts, type of workouts, different times. Three of them are cardio, five of them are toning, and two of them are stretching.

"Some of them incorporate light weights. Some of them have the exercise bands, and it's all targeted to these specifics: one targets the chest or the back, and the second one targets shoulders and arms. The third one targets hips, thighs, and buns. Each one of those is a complete ten-minute workout all on its own. There's a warmup and a cool down.

"Let's say you're used to working out in the gym. It takes one hour a day or forty-five minutes, or whatever it is. And then you can't get there one day, bad weather, schedule conflict, the kids driving you up the wall, your husband's driving you crazy—whatever it is, you can't get to the gym.

"You have ten minutes. Most of you will say, 'I can't do it today, so never mind. Forget about it; I'll do it tomorrow.' With the workout, something else happens, and before you know it, two weeks go by, you haven't done a thing, and you get miserable and don't do a thing for another year after that.

"So the nice thing about the express workout is that if you have ten minutes, at least you can do something. Maybe it's not enough as far as a workout is concerned, but it definitely gets something done. More importantly, it keeps you on track: 'You know what, I did something yesterday, so it's okay. I'll go tomorrow and do a little bit more.' So it keeps you on the wagon. It's like an emotional crutch a little bit."

Now, this is a real treat! Getting specific fitness, eating, and health advice from a world-class personal trainer and elite expert like Gilad is a bonus within a bonus! So here are Gilad's dozen elite tips for getting your own *more healthy, happy, and fit YOU*:

Top 12 Tips from Gilad

#1: To stay inspired, find a workout you can sustain. Here's the most important thing about sustainability and inspiration. A lot of people tend to make the program very difficult. Unfortunately, the trend right now is doing very intense workouts, which are not sustainable, in my opinion, except for the very few. So the most important thing for the average person just trying to do it for his own benefit and his own health and fitness is to always keep a program that he can do with ease. And when I'm saying "with ease," I don't mean he shouldn't feel sore or anything. I just mean that he knows that he can do it, and he feels good after the workout, not completely exhausted and spent, and over-the-top tired. Otherwise, you can do it for three days, or for a month, or three weeks, whatever it is, and then he'll be off the wagon again. You have to find a program that fits into your daily schedule. If you're a morning person, you do it in the morning. If you're a night person, you do it at night; whatever fits into your schedule that you know you can do.

#2: Don't make contracts in your mind that your body can't keep. You always have to find a program or workout schedule that is comfortable and easy for you to do. Of course, if you're a competitive athlete, then you have a completely different training system and program, and you have coaches, and the whole thing. But if you're an average person at home who just wants to get into better shape, wants to lose a few extra pounds from the holidays, whatever it is, the key is to always maintain a program that you can control, so that you feel fun.

#3: Don't give it all away. Never completely exhaust yourself because of the workout. Always walk away from a workout with something left.

#4: Slow and steady wins the race. Most people want the quick fix. It took them thirty years to get out of shape, or six months to gain fifteen pounds, and now they want to do it overnight. So they'll go on all these crazy low cal, no cal diets, fasts, and deprivation. And they try to fix in two weeks or a week what took them months or years to get to, and that's a really, very bad idea. Because you have to say, "Okay, I made a decision that I want to get back in shape or lose twenty to fifty pounds. I'll just do something a little bit every day and just control it and take the time to do it in a safe manner, not in a hurried and rushed manner." Those are the ones who usually fail. And the ones who usually succeed and are able to maintain their weight loss and fitness levels are the ones who ease into it, do it the right way, continue eating good, healthy foods, exercising regularly, not overdoing it, and not underdoing it, 'cause those are the ones in the long run who have the best success rate.

#5: Don't use the people on TV as your role model. Unfortunately, on a lot of programs, you see a lot of people who are 300 pounds, who need to lose 100 pounds, something like the *Biggest Loser* or something like that—it makes for good television. It doesn't make sustainability for these people. I frankly don't like the way they go about it—eliminate people that lose weight. Why would I eliminate anybody who lost weight? That will be so hard; so counterintuitive to anyone who helps people lose weight.

#6: Sweat is good for you! I've talked to a lot of people who, when I say, "Hey, let's go to the gym," they answer, "No, I don't like to sweat." So I go "okay." The sweat is actually something that helps metabolically, that helps open your pores and circulates the blood.

#7: Beware of abundance. In the United States, we have abundance of everything. So we have the best food in the world, best access to food in the world. We feed half the world off of our fields here. Some people don't know it, but we basically send rice and corn and food everywhere in the world, so we are a society of abundance. Unfortunately, it's proven through history when you have abundance, you also tend to get lazy. And then it's like bigger is better, more is better. Then you go to the movie theater, they tell you for the next $2.25 I'm going to double gulp you on the big huge – you can get a tanker instead of a cup. So people go, "Oh, yeah, I want it—the bigger the better." I just had a conversation with somebody today about something like that. They said, "No, I think bigger is better," then I –said, "No, no. Bigger is not necessarily better." So we've gotten used to this sort of abundance. And we can do whatever we want, we can eat whenever we want. We are never hungry. Twenty-four hours a day you can go and find yourself something to eat. The size of the dinner plates have doubled since the 1940s and 1950s. If you look at your parents' or grandparents' dinner plates, they were about two-thirds the size of the dinner plates today, which basically means that they have portioned. They ate less per portion. So I say the number one thing is portion and quality of your food. This is number one.

#8: Make fitness a priority. We're a very sedentary society and you really have to go out of your way to do fitness. It used to be that you would go out in the street and play with your friends. Now you can't do that anymore for a hundred different reasons. Somebody has to drive you if you're a ten- or twelve-year-old kid, or a nine-year-old kid. They have to drive you to go play.

They have to drive you back. People like to be on their computers, on their iPhones, on their technology. Their fingers do the walking, but they don't.

#9: Maintain your machine. We have these bodies; in order to work them, in order to exercise them, in order to maintain them long term, we have to maintain this machine. It's a matter of making it an important part of your life, giving it some thought, and giving it some time. I mean, I know so many people out there that if they have something material, like a nice house, they'll spend hours cleaning it and working on it. And somebody who has a really nice car will spend hours cleaning his car, fussing with his car, but sometimes when it comes to their own body, they neglect it. The body's the only thing you have for the rest of your life. You can't change it. You can't swap it. You can't trade it in. You can't lease a new one.

#10: Be proud of what's in your fridge! We would see more fruits and vegetables on our plates every single day. We would see no carbonated drinks in the refrigerator except maybe on rare occasions.

#11: It just takes a little bit of control. We are, in many ways, what we eat. So if we eat healthy, that translates into our body. The food we eat goes into the cells of the body and is broken down into the chemistry of the body. If you put junk and chemicals into your body, it affects you. The nice thing about it is that you can actually change at any time of your life. If you make a change like that, it takes maybe two or three months before you start seeing some really dramatic results. It's a matter of having a little bit of control over what you're doing, whether it's the portions or the quality of the food you eat. Jack LaLanne used to say, "If man made it, don't eat it." It's true. Take a look at pancakes. I watch people eat breakfast, and they have pancakes almost every single morning. You look at pancakes, you go, "Yes, it's very tasty but it doesn't really have much nutritional value." So if you have pancakes every day, I don't know what kind of quality of breakfast that is. If you have pancakes once a week, okay. If five or six days a week you're eating healthy, and one or two days you're not, your body can get away with it. But if you're junking eighty percent of the time, then you're a junkie.

#12: Decide to decide, then do something about it! Sometimes when you're trying to get into shape, and you haven't done anything, and you kinda feel miserable and you don't even know where to start, I'd say that, as they say, Rome was not built in a day. It takes one step at a time, and basically all you gotta do, if you have no idea what you're doing in fitness and you're able to walk, is just start walking around the block. Take a thirty-minute walk some place and just get your body going, and the rest will fall into place. You just gotta make that decision. That's the most important thing. Like I said, you can lead a horse to water; you can't force it to drink."

I wish you could talk with this wise, warm, and wonderful man to see just how generous of spirit Gilad can be!

Chapter 7

Getting (Cross) Fit
with **Heather Hodges**

"Start making some small incremental changes in your nutrition. Eat more vegetables and fruits, and lean meat, and not so many processed foods."
~ Heather Hodges

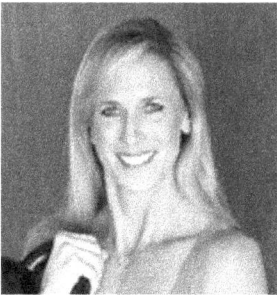

Heather Hodges is a Crossfit trainer who lives in Dallas, Texas. Many of Heather's clients prefer to begin with one-on-one training as they get started on the road to fitness.

Heather played sports in high school and volleyball in college. Then an injury sidelined both her sports and fitness goals. "Back in the early 90s," Heather explains, "I got injured in college and stopped playing ball. I had to have a couple knee surgeries. And then life happened. I got married and had children, and then one moment in my mid-thirties, I looked up and I was completely out of shape. I was soft. And I thought, *This is as good as it gets.*

"About that time, my husband Wade started going to this revolutionary new fitness program called Crossfit. I knew I had to do something about my health. I was feeling old; I was feeling tired. I knew I was too young to be feeling this old kind of feeling.

"As I watched him start to go back to the gym, he started to get into some seriously good shape. And for about three months, I just watched him and watched him, and he would come home and tell me about the workout. And I would think, *Oh my goodness, he's nuts. He's crazy! No one can work out like that!*

"Then I thought it was a fad that would blow over. Month after month, he started dropping lots of body fat, and was looking really lean and getting stronger than he'd been in our whole marriage. He fell in love with Crossfit. From his first workout, he was hooked.

"He would come home and tell me about the workout, and he'd tell me about these women who were chiseled from stone, and I thought *I am never going there. That is not for me. That sounds intimidating.* I was scared. I thought it was crazy workouts anyway. I was a college athlete. I knew how you were supposed to work out, supposedly. I knew what you're supposed to do to get results.

"And I'm watching him, getting in all this shape. And it kind of changes him along the way, and I'm thinking, *Oh, this is not going to last.* I was starting to get pretty jealous, to tell you the truth."

But once Heather decided to get involved with Crossfit, she realized she could find a home there. She explains, "Wade was actually out of town one weekend, and I called up this trainer and said, 'Okay whatever you're doing to my husband, do to me. So I had already had three training sessions with the

Crossfit trainer before he got home. I was kind of having to eat a little crow there. But I fell in love with it, too. And from the first workout, I thought, *Wow. Whatever that was, I gotta do that again.* Yeah, it was hard, and it hurt, but I was starting to see results like Wade was.

"And there is a little competitiveness to Crossfit, because every workout is timed, and it's in a class setting, so you're competing against yourself. You're trying to beat the clock. And there's also a little competitiveness with your buddy, and you want to beat your buddy, which is all in good fun.

"But that also resonated with me as a former athlete, and Wade as well. And I think that's one of the reasons he I and I just fell in love with it. It was different every day. It wasn't boring. It was hard. We learned new skills, and we got better and better and better."

Heather considers her husband, Wade, not only her partner in life but her mentor as well. "In terms of a training partner, Wade and I, we bounce things off of each other. He's probably my go-to person, my partner. In terms of fitness as well as in business, he's just brilliant. So, he's one of my favorite trainers, too."

Heather trains a wide range of people, and a large number as well; she has eighty-five to ninety clients on average. Of course, she's assisted by a strong team of Crossfit trainers.

"We train everybody at Defiant Crossfit," says Heather. "I train everybody from seven-year-olds, and I think my oldest athlete is seventy-seven. So there is a pretty broad range there. But the largest demographics are soccer moms and soccer dads, thirties to forties. These are the people who were fit at one time, and somewhere along the way they woke up and said, 'Oh my goodness, when did this happen? Where did these extra forty pounds come from? I feel tired, I feel miserable. I know something has got to change; my health is more important to me now than it was twenty years ago, so I have to make some changes.' So the majority of the people are like that."

What's great about Heather is how devoted she is to the Crossfit way of life, which as you'll find is a very specific way of training, of working out, even of thinking about fitness in general.

Heather explains, "Officially, the Crossfit is a constantly varied, functional movement performed at high intensity. What people need to know about Crossfit is that it is scalable for every level: every fitness level, every age, and every ability level. And so knowing that can help take away the intimidation of Crossfit.

"Crossfit recently teamed up with Reebok, so now it's Reebok Crossfit. So, we're working more commercials on TV featuring the best Olympic athletes in the world doing Crossfit, and you can get an impression of, 'Oh my goodness, that does look pretty scary.' But in reality, if you walk into a Crossfit gym, you're going to see a grandma training right next to a firefighter who's right next to a soccer mom while there's a Crossift kids class going on with six-, seven- and eight-year-olds.

"And what I want people to understand is that regardless of where you're coming from, regardless of your fitness background, whether you're starting from ground zero, whether you have a hundred fifty pounds to lose or five pounds to lose, Crossfit is for you, because we can scale it to your ability and take you from wherever you are and move you forward from there.

"Every Crossfit class in the world, and this is just the Crossfit model, happens in a class setting where you're with a trainer, with a coach, that is with you at all times.

"And so usually, most gyms, when you walk in, you get some information about cost, observe a class, and a lot of times they give you a free workout, so you can experience it for yourself if you want. But most Crossfit gyms will put you through a beginner class. Sometimes they call it On Ramp or Element, where the first thing you are going to do is sit down and write out your fitness goals, take a before picture, get your body fat measurements, and then you're going to set up a baseline workout fitness assessment you'll do with the trainer; then, for the remainder of that beginning class—sometimes it's a week, sometimes it's a month—you're going to learn all the elements of Crossfit: all the movements, the form, the lifts. So that when you get into class, first of all, you're not going to injure yourself because you already know the form on the lift.

"And, in our gym in particular, you have to earn your weight. What I mean by that is you have to show proficiency in a movement, in a lift, before you can put weight on a barbell. Our primary focus is safety, but our secondary focus is moving the athlete forward in terms of their fitness goals. And so people are integrated into classes, and the classes are also scalable to each athlete. So everyone in that class is going to be doing the same workout, but the load and the number of reps and the intensity is going to be scaled.

"So, let's say I have the soccer mom, Mee-maw, and firefighter in the same class. They're doing the same movements. Let's say they're doing pushups and running, and then they're doing a barbell movement, and they're doing deadlifts. All three of these people are very dramatically different athletes who are going to be doing that same workout, but with a different load, different scaling, and different intensity. Let's say the firefighter—he's going to go hard; she is going to go hard—actually, the firefighters I have in my gym are female. She's going to go hard; she's going to go intense; she'll go heavy. She's probably going to do more rounds of the workout because she's going to get through it faster. Whereas Mee-maw's going to go lighter; she's going to take her time; she'll do her pushups on the wall or on her knees.

"The soccer mom's going to go moderate weight on her dead lifts; she's going to jog and walk. She'll do some of her pushups on her knees, or she'll do some of her pushups on her toes. They're all doing the same work, but their capacity for load and reps may be different. Their needs as athletes are the same, so they'll still need to be doing the same thing.

"So our job as trainers and coaches is to know the athletes and scale the workout appropriately for their ability. Sometimes it's just encouraging them to do little more than they think they can. Sometimes it's holding them back from doing more than they need to be doing. There's usually some discussion between the coach and the athlete about how they are feeling that day. Are we going to go hard or are we going to go light? Yes, the coach is in charge of and responsible for the load and scaling of each workout for each athlete."

Heather is deeply engrained in the Crossfit lifestyle, as are her clients. She explains the whiteboard process that is so popular in the Crossfit Culture. "So, what is this whiteboard thing? It is a place where you write out the workout, but then you also record your scores every day as well.

"So when you walk into our gym, for example, when you walk into Defiant (the name of Heather's gym), a lot of people walk over to the whiteboard immediately and see what we are doing today. What torture is on the menu?

"Because every workout is different, and so we program workout, strength training, a warmup, a cool down, and it is different every single day, and so they're walking in to look at what's going to happen, what is the workout for the day, what weight are we going to be using.

"You write your name on the board, and then after the workout you write your time on the board. And so one of the things about Crossfit is that we measure, and remeasure, and check and recheck. And you can change your fitness level based on the workouts you do and how you're improving them.

"In Crossfit, there are some benchmark workouts. There are some that are named after women, and there are some that are named after fallen heroes.

"One of the most famous girl workouts is, 'Fran.' Fran is just two movements: it's a squat crunch, some people call it a squat thruster, with a barbell, and pull-ups. It is forty-five squat thrusters, and forty-five pull-ups simple, simple. But it can take the most elite athlete and put them flat on their back in two or three minutes, or it can take a soccer mom ten minutes and she'll be flat on her back.

"It is an amazing combination, and so you can look at your Fran Time, and any Crossfit athlete in the world, and they will tell you, 'This is my Fran time.' So the clock starts and we say, 'Three … two … one … Go,' and we do Fran, and we do it in seven minutes.

So you train, train, train, train, train. Three months later, six months later, you come back and do Fran again, and now it is down to three minutes—a significant drop in how much time it takes you to do that workout.

Heather never likes to see her clients "break the bank" when they come to her for training, but she also believes that fitness, like any other thing of value, is not just an event, but an investment.

"Investing in your health is investing in your future," she cautions, "and one of the things I like to help people understand when they're starting a fitness program or looking at supplementation, or whatever, is that they're already spending that money.

"I want to help people allocate that money from something that is unhealthy for them to something that is healthy for them. One of the things that Wade and I noticed when we first started Crossfitting was that we started changing our nutrition a little bit, and lo and behold, we started saving money. Because we weren't going out to eat as much, I actually kicked my Dr. Pepper habit. We weren't hitting the vending machines, or drinking a lot of fancy sodas, or fancy coffees, or anything like that. And so in terms of our overall budget, our food costs went down, and we started saving money, and we started eating healthy and not spending so much money on junk, to tell you the truth. That's part of my job as well—to help people figure out where they can trim their budget to reallocate funds toward their goal."

Heather is also a big believer in the mental and even the spiritual aspect of fitness as a lifestyle; this philosophy is instrumental when she trains others. "It helps to begin with a mission," she explains, "and understanding what motivates people to start working out in the first place, and then reminding them of that.

"That's another reason that we sit down and write out goals from the very beginning, and we keep those goals in mind when motivation starts to lag. But for sustainability, there is such a thing as overtraining, and when you train too much, your body becomes taxed, and it's hard to recover, and a whole bunch of other things start to happen metabolically, and you don't want that.

"So I try to encourage people to take it slow. We go slow at first so that we can go a long time. We're not training for the Olympics; were not training for a sprint; it's a marathon. It's for your long-term health. And so we need to find sustainability in your training, and your nutrition."

So, how do you get sustainability in your fitness lifestyle? Or, specifically, how often does Heather suggest you exercise? "What I like to see people do is to work out three times a week," she explains, "and every once in a while take some time off from that as well, whether it's going on vacation or taking a couple weeks off to let your body recover.

"But it's also important just to play, because if it's fun, you're more likely to do it and enjoy your workout. I used to think that the way you got fit was to run—and I was miserable. I had to talk myself into it every single time. Even to this day, I don't run unless I absolutely have to. Wade is the runner; he loves running. I don't like running. I like picking up heavy things."

Now it's time to let Heather share her top 12 training tips for how you can attain and keep a better body without making fitness your full-time job (that is, unless you want to).

Top 12 Tips from Heather

#1: It's okay to have fun when you're exercising. Find something you enjoy, whether it's going to play some tennis or softball. Or, some people really love yoga, or, to me, Crossfit is playtime. In fact, when I'm setting up my workout, I say, "Okay, kids, get your toys out." To me it's a lot of fun, and I enjoy it. But if you can find a workout that is enjoyable to you, you're more likely to stick with it. Some people love swimming, so get in the pool; go do something that you have fun doing.

#2: Don't do too much at once. There is the occasional person who can go cold turkey, whole hog, a 360-degree turnaround with their nutrition, and with working out. Sometimes this is sustainable, but that's kind of rare. I like to see people make incremental changes, because those seem to be more sustainable long-term. **Small changes lead to BIG results.** I don't like to see people coming in and spending a bunch of money on new workout clothes, new shoes, or whatever, at first, and then a month later they're done. I'd rather see them make small changes and start with, you know, getting to the gym two times a week, three times a week, for the next month; then we are going to tackle this, then were going to start with breakfast, then we we're going to change lunch, then we'll change snack. So these small incremental changes help people keep the good changes longer.

#3: Avoid the trap of overtraining. I see that with even a lot of Crossfitters who love, love, love Crossfit, and they train hard, but then they keep getting these old nagging injuries. Their shoulder is bothering them, their knee is bothering them, and they don't take time off to recover; then, they fall into the overtraining trap. One of the most elite athletes that I have had the privilege of training was training for Crossfit games last year, which is kind of like the Olympics of Crossfit. She was Crossfitting several times a day. She was in the top thirty Crossfitters in the world. And then all of a sudden, she started feeling really bad. As it turned out, she had adrenal failure, which is stress on her system, and it took a while to come back from that. She was overtraining, over stressing her body. And so she was forced to sit down and not train for a little while.

#4: Your body needs rest. You get stronger when you rest, not when you're lifting weights. Your body absolutely has to rest. A lot of type-A people want to train hard. They also are high stress at work, high stress in their private life, and maybe they're not sleeping eight or nine hours a night like they need to be doing, and they just tax their body too much—and it's basically overstressing the body.

#5: Don't let being a mom get in the way of being all that you can be. The person that I have in mind is a mom, she has small children, and she has a real situation, but she does not have the time to work out; she does not have childcare, and she uses the isolation of being a stay-at-home mom as an excuse not to exercise. When the kids are little, it's hard to get out of the house, and we moms tend to give, give, give, give, give, and we don't spend any time on ourselves, we neglect ourselves. But if she would spend a little bit, a couple hours a week, just on herself, that's not being selfish. I have even talked to other mothers who have said, 'I just don't feel led to do that right now because it would be selfish of me.' But they would be better moms, better spouses, better examples for their family, because they would have more energy, and their moods would get better, and they would be setting such a big example of health and wellness and fitness for their children, and even for their husbands. A lot of times it's moms who lead the way back to fitness, and if I could get her to just start training and working out just a little bit, I know she'd feel better, and she'd have more energy, and do the things that she feels like she doesn't have the energy to do right now, for her kids.

#6: Stop buying bigger clothes. At some point, you have to stop buying bigger and bigger clothes. It starts to get really expensive. And you look in the mirror and say, "How on earth did this happen?"

#7: Skip the sugar. I would encourage everybody to put the sugar down and walk away. It is so prevalent in our society, and in our culture in particular, in our food and drink. I would say drink more water and less sugar.

#8: Start small, but start somewhere. Start making some small incremental changes in your nutrition. Eat more vegetables and fruits, and lean meat, and not so many processed foods. You do not have to drive through McDonald's. That is not your only option for yourself, or for your children.

#9: Go outside and play. Do something you enjoy doing instead of just sitting. Go play with your children, go play with the dog, go do something that you enjoy. Chances are you're more likely to lose a little weight and start feeling a little bit better, your energy will increase, and your mood is going to be better.

#10: Family first. I would hope that families would start eating dinners together instead of just grabbing drive–through meals. This would help keep families together and talking to each other, and being a part of each other's lives in general, instead of just grabbing take-out whenever they can.

#11: Patient, heal thyself. In terms of health, we would stop having to visit the doctor so much if we ate healthy foods and exercised more. A lot of the illnesses in our country are directly related to our nutrition, or lack thereof. I mean, looking at diabetes and heart disease, even cancer, some of the cancer we're seeing now is directly related to nutrition.

#12: Don't neglect the spiritual aspect of why we train. There's a very holistic quality to training, getting back in shape, and disciplining ourselves in terms of eating and training. We can't separate who we are in Christ with how we eat, how we train, how we treat our children, and how we do business. To us, it's all the same, so I like to incorporate that as well. Sit down and write out your physical goals, spiritual goals, and performance goals, and all of these things are going to come together to help make you a more well-rounded you, a more complete holistic you, as a child of God, as a mom, as a wife, as an employee, as whatever— all these things are going work together, and we don't train for the sake of ourselves. Yeah, it's great to fit into a bikini, but that's not what it's about. We train for the sake of others. We train so that we can be a better mom and a better wife. We train so that we can rescue our children when they run into the middle of the road—that's why we train. We train for ourselves, but we train for others.

Thanks, Heather, for sharing your personal and professional views on what it takes to get and keep your better body!

Chapter 8

Be a Turtle, Not a Hare
with **Lindsay Wright**

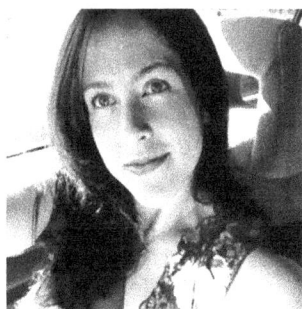

"The people who succeed are more turtle-like than rabbit-like, because when the rabbit types take too much on, they put their hands up and say, 'That's enough. It's not worth it.'"
~ Lindsay Wright

Lindsay Wright runs "Lindsay's List," a popular healthy living blog, where she shares lists that she's working on. You'll find workouts, recipes, bad jokes, and adorable kids. Her readers love her!

Lindsay also wears MANY hats! A loving wife to Travis and mother to toddlers Henry and Clara, Lindsay also teaches step, water aerobics, and boot camp classes, and works as a personal trainer. As an NASM-certified trainer, Lindsay creates custom fitness regimens for weight-loss clients and athletes.

An avid runner, Lindsay's fitness philosophy is "Get out and MOVE!" Her hobbies include singing as part of her church's worship team, clipping coupons, eating under-baked brownies, and catching up on fitness blogs.

Lindsay is a certified personal trainer and group fitness instructor at Franklin Health and Fitness Center in Franklin, North Carolina, which is about an hour west of Asheville.

Like many of the trainers we've spoken with for *Better Body Wannabe*, Lindsay's first experiences in the health field began at a young age. She explains, "I've always been into fitness, even from a young age, just doing sports such as basketball, track, and cross-country running. When I was in cross-country in high school, I developed an eating disorder, which lasted into college, and those were some rough years. I came out of the eating disorder with the help of my husband and just wanted to direct that toward helping other people, whether in fitness or food, and that's how I got involved."

Much as Lindsay credits her husband with helping her through her eating disorder, she credits chance for getting her working in the fitness field in the first place.

She explains, "When we first got married, we moved out to Colorado, and I worked in a gym because I wanted a membership there, but I didn't want to pay for it. (When you work in a gym, you usually get free membership.) That was just a monthly expense that we didn't have to pay for, so that's kind of what started it."

From there, Lindsay found that she had a passion for helping others, and she put it to use in the gym. The drive to change and help others change is what started her long career in fitness. That and seeing "… food as fuel instead of something bad, or something that we should neglect our bodies with."

One of the perks of working in a gym is that Lindsay can bring her two children with her. "It's a great career for anybody who wants to be a mom, because you can set your own hours, and most gyms have daycares. I have two children, and they come to the gym with me. If anything happens, I'm right there, and we've had that happen before where I've had to step out of a class. But it's just reassuring to know that they're right there."

It's a good thing, too, because from the sound of it, Lindsay is at the gym a LOT. "Every week I teach beginners step aerobics," she explains. "I teach boot camp classes, and I teach aqua aerobics. They're all sixty-minute classes at my gym, and I train clients as well."

What type of regimen does Lindsay personally use? "I aim for five days of exercise, two days of rest," she explains. "I usually teach a class every day. So I teach sixty minutes of exercise there. If I'm not teaching, I love lifting weights, and I usually do circuit training with about a ten-minute warm-up and a circuit of either total body, upper body, or lower body, and then I try to do about twenty minutes of intense interval work either on the treadmill or elliptical."

When it comes to inspiration, Lindsay doesn't have to look too far from home. "Personally, my husband inspires me every day. He lifted with me in college. He introduced me to the weight room. I was a cardio buddy for a long time, and he's the one who got me into the weight room."

As a mother of two, Lindsay is particularly empathetic to new mothers seeking to shed their baby weight. She also comes armed with dual certifications to help them do just that!

"I have certifications in pre- and post-natal training," she explains, "so I do focus a lot of my attention and marketing on new moms who want to get their pregnancy weight off because I've been there and done it twice. And I have clients who are pregnant or have just been pregnant."

Lindsay always gets excited when she can help her clients meet, or even exceed, their weight loss goals. "Every twelve weeks we run a weight loss challenge. And we have probably about twenty participants every challenge. They get to train with a client at the gym two times a week, and then we give them a nutrition plan. I think our last winner lost about sixty or sixty-five pounds within twelve weeks!"

Lindsay personally trains about seven clients a week, and is usually at the gym on average about three hours a day, training. When it comes to weight loss, Lindsay favors interval training. "We do kind of a three-minute approach," she explains. "We do a strength training move for a minute, and then we do a plyometric move for a minute, and then I do a sprint for a minute, and then we rest for a minute.

"I usually try to do compound movements—like a squat with a bicep curl, or a squat with an overhead press. Then we do a plyometric move such as jump squats, or jumping jacks, or wall jumps. And then we get on the treadmill, and I have them sprint for a minute, and then we rest for a minute, and then we do that all over again.

"I like that format, and my clients love it, because you can do anything for a minute. And they know that rest is coming in three minutes, so that's a great approach."

So, what are some of Lindsay's favorite tips for getting that better body in a way that won't put her clients in traction? Here are twelve of her favorite ideas:

Top 12 Tips from Lindsay

#1: Don't do too much too soon. I think the mistake that a lot of people fall into is they try to do too much too quickly. They'll be in the gym every day trying to do something. And I really tell clients to try to—when you're just starting, try to get in there three times a week. Anybody can get in there three times a week. If you can do more than that, great.

#2: Rest is critical. I always say to take one day of full rest, if not two. The people who succeed are more turtle-like than rabbit-like, because when the rabbit types take too much on, they put their hands up and say, "That's enough. It's not worth it." So studies state just keep packing away at it, and if you feel a little overwhelmed, step back, go back to your three days a week, and then come back.

#3: Breaks can be beneficial. Most of my clients do take a holiday, and they won't work out at all. But a lot of them see vacation as a way to change up their work-outs, so they don't necessarily do the same strength or cardio plan. But they go for daily walks on the beach, or they try to incorporate movement into their vaca-tion, like taking hikes or going sightseeing. There are ways that you can do that, and you can do a ton of stuff just in your hotel room with resistance bands and body weights movements.

#4: Find your niche, and the passion will follow. I think a lot of people who don't like to exercise just haven't found the exercise that fits their personality. I think a lot of people who might give up too quickly just haven't found their little niche in the workout arena. So maybe try out different classes or different machines at the gym that you haven't tried out before, or try working out with a partner and having that accountability—things like that.

#5: Pick the right kind of class for you. If you are very competitive, you need to be in boot camp class. If you like to come to the gym and zone out, and not think about what you're doing, maybe a spinning class is good. There's no talking. You just do what the instructor says.

#6: Take your injuries seriously. If you have injuries, you need to be in the pool.

#7: Get hydrated. My clients don't drink enough water. Water is free. Everyone can drink water, and it has no calories. I'll ask all my clients how much water they're drinking, and maybe they get half of what is recommended. I drink about 120 ounces of water a day, and it just helps in so many ways. It helps digestion. It helps you feel full. It helps keep your skin clear, and it helps hydrate your body for working out.

#8: Start a weight-lifting program. Weight lifting has a myriad of benefits, but a lot of women, in particular, don't take it up because they think they're going to get bulked up or they're going to gain weight. They're scared to step into the weight room with all the guys. Start a weight-lifting program.

#9: Build movement into your day. Whether it be parking farther away at the grocery store or taking the stairs, create little windows of opportunity for movement, such as getting out of your desk chair to get water on the next floor and different things like that. We burn the least amount of calories sitting down; even just choosing to stand up more often makes a difference. I think that would help a lot.

#10: Remember that exercise and getting fit are so much more mental than physical. There are so many physical benefits of exercise, but the mental benefits are just huge. It's been proven that when you exercise, your body releases mood-lifting endorphins, so you feel better about yourself and about situations. When you feel better about yourself, you approach others with an improved idealism, so you view relationships in a better light. It's a whole wellness approach to life, eating, drinking water, getting enough sleep, having a better sex life, exercising, all of those things. It's all like a circle. So exercise is just one piece of this whole puzzle.

#11: Find a trainer who inspires you. I don't like barky, "drop and give me twenty" kinds of trainers. I like motivational trainers.

#12: Just get started. It's so not that hard. Even if you can just do twenty minutes of something every day, it will vastly improve everything: your outlook on life, your body, your relationships, your mental health, your physical health. Just get started.

Thanks, Lindsay, for sharing your time with us and offering us these twelve life-altering tips!

Chapter 9

Less Is More
with Thomas "Doc" Masters

"You have to have things that you like to do. I don't care if it's flying kites, miniature golfing, and whatever you like to do, you have to do things."
~ "Doc" Masters

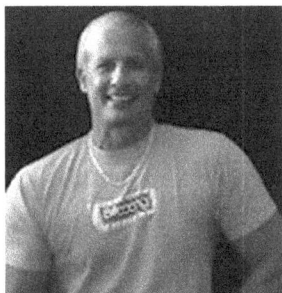

Thomas "Doc" Masters is the founder of Flex-Appeal. Flex-Appeal is a premier accomplished personal training company located in Dana Point, California. Workouts consist of a personalized combination of TRX, Pilates, plyometrics, balance, core exercises, and FUN!

Lots of people wonder where the nickname Doc came from. "Well," Doc explains, "I was dubbed Doc by my sailing crew when I was a racing sailor, tending to the many bumps, bruises, strains, and sprains of my fellow crewmembers. I have been a competitive athlete and trainer for over twenty years."

Like many of the trainers interviewed for this book, fitness seems to be in Doc's blood. He explains, "This has been a life-long thing for me. I've been an athlete my whole life. I was an athlete back in college; it's what I have my degree in. I can't think of anything else I'd rather do, really. I've never been out of shape. I love fitness. I love getting people healthy."

Doc calls his personal brand of training active exercise or Active X. He clarifies, "It's a combination of Pilates, plyometrics, heavy-duty core work, balance work, a lot of sports drills from different sports that I've worked at, and just a real lot of combinations that all add up to you being more functional."

Doc's attitude about his clients is one of change, innovation, and flow. "I change it up," he explains, "so you never know what I'm coming up with that day. I do my homework every night depending on who I'm going to train the next day, and I make up their program. I change it every week so that they never know what they'll be doing every week. And I might throw in a few things that they've already done, because you can only gauge how good someone's getting if they're doing something that they've already done.

"When it comes right down to it, the confusion is what keeps them healthy. It's all about being healthy now. It's not about gaining the advantage or just having a good-looking body. But the types of workouts that we're doing now do make you strong, and they do give you endurance, and they do make you more healthy."

Doc uses simplicity in his workouts, but also to show clients how out of shape they may be. "It just makes it easier to teach," he says. "It just makes it more fun. When somebody does something that's really simple and they can't do it, it's really easy for them to see how out of shape they are. When you tell someone to pick a ball up, turn around, sit down, pick a ball up, turn around, sit down, and they can do that, they sit down and say, 'Oh, man, I'm out of shape. Even little kids can do this.' It really motivates people that way."

When asked about any fitness mentors that may have molded or shaped his career or beliefs about the fitness industry, one name leaps to mind. "Some of the very earliest memories I have in my life are my mother with her 50's hair exercising to Jack LaLanne on the black-and-white television," Doc recalls fondly. "That was just so motivating to me, and that man lived so long, he walked his talk through his whole life.

"Jack lived the straight life, exercised, and was always motivated. That's what I'd like to do. I'm almost fifty-seven. It works; it really works. It doesn't mean you have to live a certain lifestyle. It doesn't mean you can never have fun; it means you got to do things in moderation."

Doc's clientele is wide and varied, but the clients that are particularly close to his heart are those near the end of their lives. "I have a couple contracts with care facilities," he explains. "I work more with people who have one foot in the grave. I'm their big deal for the week when I come in. I have a lot of fun with them, too.

"It's kind of sad to watch people get old and get pushed around. Nobody listens to them, and they're heavily medicated. It's kind of a sad thing to think that we might all end up like that ultimately."

With his regular clients, Doc has a holistic attitude about fitness, and insists that whatever you do, it must be sustainable but also fun. "What's going to make you stay fit is to have recreational activities that you do," he insists. "You have to have things that you like to do. I don't care if it's flying kites, miniature golfing, and whatever you like to do, you have to do things."

This type of workout, Doc explains, is extremely conducive to working out with others, particularly whole families working out together. "The families that I train that do things together are the good strong families because they have fun. They work together, they compete against each other, and they spend time together. That's important for families. It doesn't matter what activity you do, but that gives you a reason to work out."

As one might imagine, Doc has some very specific advice on how to achieve a better body, and I think you'll find his top 12 fitness, weight loss, and overall health tips both fascinating and illuminating on your own journey to wellness.

Top 12 Tips from Doc

#1: Fitness takes time. A journey of a thousand miles starts with one step. Put one foot in front of the other and keep doing it. That's all there is to it. And if you do that, one day you will wake up and be fit. You'll eat right because it's the right thing to do, because you don't want to eat crap food anymore. Then when you look at people who eat badly, you'll feel sorry for them, and then you'll think, *Why would I ever want to eat that?* You won't once you know what's in it. The easiest thing for me is when they come back to me when they have been training with me for a while, and they say, "I don't even drink anymore. I don't like to drink anymore. I don't like to have a hangover." Or, "I don't like eating saturated fat foods anymore. I can't even look at that bag of Cheetos, and I used to eat them every day. I feel sorry for people who drink soda; it's so bad for you." And that's when I tell them, "Yes! You got it!"

#2: You are who you hang around with. All my friends are really fit; all my clients are really fit. I just hang around a lot of really active people. I don't know anybody who's really close to me who is inactive in some way. I really don't. My dad was an athlete his whole life. My mom was a smoker for years, and then she quit. Everybody around me is pretty fit.

#3: Don't eat anything that's in a box. Don't eat anything that's in a package. Eat whole foods. It's the most important thing in life. Fruits, vegetables, meat—eat anything that's whole. Don't eat genetically-modified foods, which means canola, corn, and soy. Stay away from those things. You have to. They're terrible. They're poison.

#4: You have to stay away from high fructose corn syrup. High fructose corn syrup will rot your liver.

#5: You have to stay away from artificial sweeteners like aspartame. It's poison. Anything that has artificial flavor in it is poison. There's only one way to get that artificial flavor, and that's through chemicals that simulate that flavor. All you're eating is chemicals.

#6: Stay away from table salt. Table salt contains sodium chloride, which is a chemical. When you take table salt into your body, your body does not want it there, so it surrounds it with water so that you can get it out of your body by urinating it out. And by doing that, it pulls all the water from the surrounding cells and kills them. And that's why your blood pressure goes up. People who want to salt their food should use sea salt or kosher salt because those have all the minerals that belong in your body, because your body is saltwater. You're 98 percent water. We need salt.

#7: Kosher is kosher. When in doubt, eat kosher food because it's not altered; there are no fillers—it is against their religion. And they're really tight on enforcing that. They don't mess around with that stuff.

#8: Chlorine is a poison. In order to make water clean they have to use chlorine in the filtration system, because if they didn't there would be so many bacteria in the water that we'd die. As the end user, you need to filter out that chlorine. When you take a fifteen- or twenty-minute shower, it's like drinking about eight or ten glasses of chlorinated water—and nobody drinks chlorinated water anymore. All you need is a cheap thirty-dollar filter on your shower and change it out once a year, or whatever the manufacturer recommends, and then you don't have the chlorine.

#9: Stop drinking bottled water! People drink bottled water like it's going out of style. What people don't understand is that bottled water has absolutely no regulation whatsoever. They can put whatever they want in bottled water. You should filter your own water so that you know you're drinking good, clean water. Your local water company that sells water through your tap is much more regulated than the companies that sell bottled water. If the water plant in your town breaks down, or if the bacteria count is too high, they close it down, and they put it in the paper, and they tell people, "Hey, don't drink the water because the water is messed up." But if that happens in the plant that's doing bottled water, they don't tell anybody about it. They don't have to. The only reason that I know these types of things is because I've done the research. I've written articles on all these things. I really know the background on this stuff.

#10: Don't try to get fit in a week. It's not about running or popping a diet pill; it is changing your lifestyle.

#11: All change is good. Keep in mind that all change is good. All change is always good, no matter what. You may not like it, you may not see the good right away, but if it's change, it's good. You're going to learn more, you're going to do new things, and meet new people.

#12: By learning, we teach. By teaching, we learn. Once you know it, you'll teach other people; you won't hold it back. It's like a little gem you have to share with everybody else. It's good. You won't be able to hold yourself back.

As always, I continue to be amazed at the variety, intensity, and sincerity of these tips from the world's best trainers, and Doc's are no exception! I'll let Doc leave you with his words of wisdom about how he treats fitness as a lifestyle, and not a job: "It's really not my job; it's my life. It's not a job for me. It's what I do. It is me; is what I am. I don't ever see me retiring from that. I teach fitness. It's what I've done my whole life, and I don't see myself retiring from that."

Those are words we can all live by, I'm sure!

Chapter 10

Working from the Inside Out
with **Tamilee Webb**

"You will keep doing it if you love it. If you don't love it, don't do it, because you know exercise and fitness will be equated with misery and duty, and that's not a good combination for a lifetime."

~ Tamilee Webb

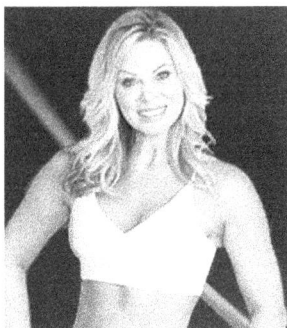

Tamilee Webb earned a bachelor of arts degree in physical education and a master of arts degree in exercise science, both attained at California State University, Chico.

She has furthered her education through involvement in IDEA, AFAA, ACE, and FROG'S Athletic Club, and is now founder and CEO of Webb International, Inc.

In 1993, Tamilee was recognized by her peers as the Fitness Instructor (Trainer) of the Year, an award bestowed by IDEA, the association of fitness professionals, after having been a three-time nominee in the category. In 1992, she received the coveted *Self* magazine award for best lower body exercise for her third in a series of twenty-two award-winning *Buns of Steel* videos.

Tamilee has been the recipient of numerous other awards for outstanding achievement in the field of personal fitness, including Best Exercise Video and Best Training Organization 1987, conferred by IDEA, and was honored by California State University, Chico, as an outstanding alumna in 1990 and 1996.

Millions of fans worldwide have long admired Tamilee's no-nonsense approach to achieving health and fitness within one's home. Her energy, exuberance, and specially designed, proven weight-loss workout programs have consistently elevated her to the top of the *Billboard* charts.

She has written four best-selling books: *The Original Rubber Band Workout* (sold in six countries and translated into five languages), *Step-up Fitness*, *Workout for Dummies*, and *Defy Gravity Workout*, all of which have contributed to the renown that she has so deservedly earned.

Tamilee has been a co-host on the Health Network Channel's aerobic fitness shows now known as Discovery's FitTV. The network serves more than fifty million households, and its audience is growing rapidly. She has also hosted ESPN's Fitness Pro Series, and consulted on Fox Sports Fitness show *Body Squad*. Tamilee is best known for her Buns of Steel series, which has sold more than ten million copies and includes her Quick-Toning Series, and she has co-hosted the Buns of Steel Platinum Series.

Tamilee's knowledge and acquired experience, combined with her contagious energy and effervescent personality, have made her an ideal guest speaker on top-rated television talk shows, including VH1's *Booty Call*, NBC's *Weekend Today*,

Entertainment Tonight, KTLA Morning News, *The Today Show*, *The Other Half, Home Matters, E! Entertainment*, and *The BIG Idea* on CNBC. Her well-toned body has graced the covers of *Shape* magazine, and *Fitness* magazine, and she has been featured in *Fit Magazine, Men's Fitness, Vogue, American Fitness*, and *Billboard*.

Tamilee realizes the impact that she has on those who rely on her to maintain and improve their health and fitness, and she takes her responsibility seriously. Her videos are released to the public only after having undergone extensive scientific testing and research as to their safety and effectiveness. She is always aware of the fact that her exercise programs are followed by people with different body types and varying levels of fitness.

With this in mind, products and equipment receive her endorsements only after serious scrutiny of their quality and results. Seen on her most recent infomercial is one of her newest and approved finds, the Ab-Away Pro abdominal exercise machine.

Although Tamilee is world renowned for her line of videos and DVDs, her progression into an elite physical trainer began quite naturally. "My father played semi-pro baseball when he was young," she explains, "and I had brothers and no sister, so I was always a little tomboy and had to play with my brothers. So I only had one doll in my entire life, and I named her Pebbles.

"I realized I really loved being fit and being active. As I got older, and when it was time for me to decide which career direction I'd go in, I thought maybe nursing because I like helping people, but I didn't really like the blood aspect of it. I realized that I also enjoy dance and music; that was my other passion. I actually thought that I was going to grow up to be the next Shania Twain, but I realized that fitness was my real true heart, and being able to help people feel good in their bodies was what I decided to go forward and do.

"When I started, aerobic dance was just coming out. I got my undergraduate degree in physical education to become a teacher; and then, in my last year, they offered exercise science, and that gave me the ability to go for my master's in that field, which today they call kinesiology. So that's kind of what led me there, but as far as videos, I just realized that once I started helping people, I could help more people if I was on television or did videos to reach a greater population."

So, how does Tamilee retain her own better body? "Well," she says, "I still get somewhat of a workout from teaching, although it's not about my workout, it's about my students' workout. But I try to mix it up. I hike with some girlfriends at least once or twice a week. I try to get in some yoga. I try to do some salsa dancing. I always try to mix things up where I'm doing something for me."

Like all the trainers we've talked to, Tamilee has a wide fan base but tends to see a specific group more than the rest. "I would say my biggest demographic is probably women age thirty-five and up," she explains. "That's the majority of my group X classes that purchase DVDs. However, I do have a fairly good following of men who buy my Abs of Steel. They still buy that product. And I would say that all my clients range anywhere from where they need to lose probably ten pounds up to seventy-five pounds."

Tamilee keeps a busy schedule and teaches, on average, anywhere from 60 to 70 people a week. You might be surprised by Tamilee's theory on the origins of health. "My philosophy is that fitness begins on the inside and work its way out. Many times we see something and say, 'That's what I want,' or 'I want abs like that,' or 'I want a body like that,' and really it's about your internal health. So I always say that if you could unzip your body and take a look on the inside, what would it look like? What would it represent?"

Tamilee considers health a gift. "The greatest thing that we could ever have is our health, because if you don't have your health, you don't have a whole lot of other things. You can't do things; you can't take care of your family, and you can't take care of you, your pets, or your home. You can't do all those wonderful things that you want to do with your friends and family, and so health is just—to me, it's the top of the list, so it starts from within."

Speaking of health, taking it slow and steady seems to be Tamilee's philosophy, particularly with beginners. "If somebody's used to eating maybe three thousand calories a day, I'm going to gradually take them down from there. So probably for the first week or two, we'll take out 200 of those calories, so we could get them down to the right amount of calories and then staying with their fitness."

One of Tamilee's pet peeves is short-term fitness goals with no habitual behavior in sight. She explains, "If they say, 'Oh, I've got this wedding to go to and I want to look really good 'cause my boyfriend's going to be there, blah, blah, blah, and I've got ten days to do it, I'm like, 'Well, good luck with that.' Because what you're going to do in ten days will come back to you with double the force because you can't necessarily lose weight in ten days and think that you're going to keep it off. You can lose it, but that doesn't mean that you're going to keep it off."

What's your most important piece of workout equipment? You might be surprised by Tamilee's answer. "Well, first of all, you should invest in a good pair of workout shoes. Because if that is the biggest investment you can afford, you can now take your body out and start walking and not get blisters."

In order to encourage healthy habits that last a lifetime, Tamilee suggests starting out slow to stay on track. "You've got to take it easy," she insists. "You can't just start off the way everybody does in the beginning of a new year. They start off, and lots of people in my classes say, 'Oh, it's crowded.' I say, 'Give it two weeks.' Unfortunately, a lot of them have dropped out because they get in there and then they get sore. It's like they just stepped on the gas pedal and away they went instead of gradually building it up."

Tamilee insists that our bodies were designed to move, and that any movement is good movement. "It's a lifestyle, not something you do for the short term. So even if you do ten minutes or you just put on your running shoes and go outside and walk or jog, if you get in twenty minutes, ten minutes— anything—your body responds. And when you don't respond, your body responds to your not responding. You take care of your body, and your body will take care of you."

As one might expect, a trainer of Tamilee's caliber has some surefire tips for getting and keeping that better body.

Top 12 Tips from Tamilee

> **#1: Do what's right for you.** I encourage people that if you never exercise and you want to get out there, let's first find the right type of activity for you. Do you prefer to be outside or inside? Do you prefer water, air, or something else? Then I know whether to get them outside or inside, and if they like being outside, do they like the water? Okay, then let's do a beach walk. Or, if they like to be inside and they enjoy dancing, then

let's do a dance class. It doesn't have to be what the greatest thing is, so if you love dancing—and Zumba is so big right now—then get into a Zumba class. You'll dance, you'll laugh, and you won't even realize that you're working out because you're having fun. And if fitness is not fun, if you don't find an activity that is fun or engaging, you're not going to stick with it. You have to find something motivating and fun that makes you want to go. Like my mom—she's got arthritis, she's got a bad knee, but she loves gardening. She's got a big yard, and even though she probably could use some help, I know that as long as she can get outside each day and keep moving her body by working in that garden, she's doing something.

#2: Fight boredom. You've got to mix it up in order to keep your body guessing. You have to change up your workout. If the same thing isn't working anymore, change it up. I did this once with a girlfriend. One day she told me what we were going to do for a workout, and the next day I told her what we were going to do. It wasn't all the same thing. So the next day, she said, "Hey, guess what? We're rollerblading today." "We are?" I said. "Okay." So we mix it up, and it is fun to do this because you're always guessing.

#3: You can make diets work if you do the work—and stick with them. Diets work if you stick with them, but if you don't plan on sticking with them, then the weight is going to creep back on. That's because your body has to make that change and stay at the new weight for a year or so in order for it to say, "Okay, we'll stay here."

#4: If you don't make time for health and fitness now, you will make time for illness later. We have to make time for things. If we don't, there's never going to be time.

#5 Listen to your body. (It listens to you!) Your body will take notice. The minute you start doing something good for your body, your body will say, "Oh, wow, look what she's doing. Okay, we'll help her out a little bit, but you know she's going to quit." And that's a gland called the hypothalamus. Now, the hypothalamus does stuff in our brain; it's kind of like the mother lode up there along with our hormones, and if you look at it as a scale, you would push that needle all the way up to where you are now, and it doesn't want to budge; it doesn't want to come back down. But if you keep at it, eventually it says, "Wow, she is serious about this. She's been doing it for a while. Okay, we'll budge a little bit." But you see, if you keep doing it and you do it too fast it says, "Okay, we're going to lose for you, but we're not going to lose the stuff that you need to lose. We're going lose muscle, which you don't want to lose, and a little bit of fat. So that way if you are really trying to starve yourself, we have enough fat to sustain your life." And then you go back to your old habits, and it says, "Okay, now let's go back to where we were, and let's add some more just in case she decides to do this again to us."

#6: A little means a lot. That's why it's important to do it a little at a time. It's like a pregnancy. When you get pregnant, it's a gradual thing. And that's kind of what our bodies do, too. It's a gradual thing, so if you've been overweight for most of your life, don't expect that you're going to be where you want to be in six weeks, twelve weeks, or even a year. And most people want to be where they were in high school or college, and that's not going to happen. Our bodies change as we get older, and we get heavier. However, we want to be fit from the inside out, and that's why I always tell people, "Okay, so you think you're skinny, but you can be skinny fat." You could be. I mean you're skinny, but let's go look and see how much of that is muscle and how much of that is fat.

#7: Start with a positive affirmation. Say good things about yourself, like, "Good morning, beautiful. We're going to have a great day. I love those arms. Look at those arms." Instead of beating ourselves up, and that's what we do, we need to start being kind and positive, and when we start loving our body mentally and emotionally, everything else will follow. But if you're beating yourself up all the time, you're just sending negative messages and energy to yourself, and that's not what anybody wants.

#8: Educate yourself. Educate yourself about you. What is it that your body responds to and doesn't? For instance, a lot of people can't eat food that is high in gluten, and it could be certain little things that you're eating that are making your digestive system not process food the way it should when you're trying to lose weight. So track your food intake and see how many grams of protein, carbs, and fats you're eating. So when you take a look at that and you go, "Wow, that's what I ate this whole day?" And find out how many calories you should need.

So let's say the average woman should eat 1,500 to 2,000 calories, and all of a sudden—and I know that they offer this now in coffee shops and various places—when you see how many calories are in the food you're about to order, do you really want it? Maybe you can split it with a friend. So it's about educating yourself of what's going into your body.

#9: Your body is meant to move. I don't care what you do to move it. If it's just putting your iPod on or turning on the music in your house and dancing around, do it. Do something. If you have a dog, I hope you're walking it. I mean, our dogs are becoming almost as obese as we are because we feed them bad food and we don't exercise them.

#10: Give fitness a chance. You're happier, your blood pressure is going down, and your anxiety and stress are going down; that's what fitness does. And all you have to do is just try it. I mean, what's the worst that can happen? Oh, you feel better, you look better, and you might even lose a few pounds.

#11: Give yourself 84 days. I have a program called E84. The E stands for Evolve, and the 84 stands for 84 days. And that's how you need to look at it. So in the first 42 days, you're going to notice the difference; the last 42 days, the world is going to recognize the difference. And that's typically how long it takes for our bodies to really start to get it and respond.

WORKING FROM THE INSIDE OUT

#12: Know your goals. When you're going to start something, and especially in fitness, is your goal just to be healthy? Is your goal to fit into a smaller size? Determine what your goal is and how you're going to get there, and then get there having fun doing it. So if it was not fun, you are going to go backwards, and you're not going to stick with it.

BONUS #13: Find a good fit with your trainer. If you need someone to yell at you and scream at you, then that might be your style. I mean, I get people who say, "I just love it 'cause you always say please," and I'm like, "I do?" And I realized I do: "Four more, please. Come on, we can do this." Everybody has a different style, so fine, if you are going to work out and train with a trainer, interview them and find out how they train. Their method may not be your style. You might need to be really pushed, so if that's the case, then you need that drill sergeant.

A special thanks to Tamilee for her insight and expertise as we all seek our own better body with the help of these great trainers, coaches, and all-around inspiring individuals.

Chapter 11

Getting Your "Beach Body"
with **Kelli Buzzard**

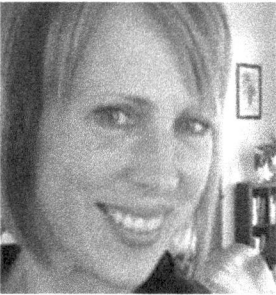

"You will keep doing it if you love it. If you don't love it, don't do it; otherwise, you will equate exercise and fitness with misery and duty, and that's not a good combination for a lifetime."
~ Kelli Buzzard

Several years ago, Kelli's sister and brother-in-law got up off the couch, ordered the world-famous P90X workout, and became ridiculously fit. When she found out that the "secret" to their success was that they simply stopped eating junk and did a ninety-day P90X challenge, she got turned on to the workout, too.

Thus began Kelli's relationship with P90X and the beginning of a journey that would lead her into fitness and nutrition coaching and much, much more.

Today, Kelli Buzzard is a Beachbody coach, and her passion for fitness, nutrition, and overall health has only grown. She also runs Fit Club workouts in her Northwest Washington community in the Skagit Valley.

Says Kelli of her new, fit self, "I am happy to say that I am as fit as I was back in my competitive sports days, and I am having way more fun! In fact, in some ways I am more fit now than I was back then: less prone to injury and sickness and more freed-up to do other things in life. In college, I did two practices each day plus two hours of weight training every day. Now, I work out thirty to seventy-five minutes a day, five days a week, and have lots of time for other interests. It's truly amazing."

As a lifelong educator, having taught middle school and currently teaching college students, Kelli has always had the coaching bug. She loves coming alongside people and helping them identify—and then reach—their goals. She has found that this desire has only increased since becoming a Beachbody coach.

Kelli explains, "Now I coach people in fitness and some in business who really want to learn, grow, and change—not always a combination you find in middle school or college students! It is highly rewarding."

Another one of Kelli's passions has always been food. She grew up in a home where healthy, fresh, local, and home-cooked food was valued. Her mom was a natural cook and passed that on to Kelli and her sister. They loved cooking—and cooking together. Not surprisingly, they have all worked together as personal chefs.

"It's such a hoot to bring joy to people by feeding them," Kelli says, "and feeding them *well*. It's also a big hoot to make foods that are healthy and that taste fantastic. One of my goals is to eat like a queen every day both in terms of nutrition and taste."

Recently Kelli expanded her food knowledge by becoming a NESTA-certified fitness nutrition coach. She loves discovering how the human body works and how nutrition plays a role in proper body functioning and physical fitness.

Kelli blogs about food, usually highlighting recipes that are shared with family and friends. She enjoys counseling her clients to maximize their training results and food enjoyment through preparing healthy, easy recipes for themselves and their families. Kelli recently began a primal or paleo eating journey (with clear results), and especially enjoys sharing classic recipes that she has paleo-ized.

Kelli grew up with sports. She says, "Growing up, I was always into sports. In fact, my dad was a really great athlete. He was very well known for his track and field, and so I sort of had that sports thing in my blood. And I grew up in a small community where most kids went out for the teams and had a chance to play sports even if we weren't the best at it. So I played sports all seasons from an early age and was a basketball player in high school, and I also played for a small college. So, basically, training was a part of my life from when I was a child."

Kelli is passionate about what that training taught her. "I wish I had known then what I know now about certain aspects of training. Over the years, different fad diets come and go, and different training philosophies and regimens come and go as well.

"Not all of them are as effective as others. When I played basketball, we did two practices a day, each a couple hours long, and then I worked with weights on my own for about two hours, so I was hard-core into working out. And I was on a low-fat diet, whenever I could get low-fat foods from our college cafeteria.

"So I wasn't getting enough protein, and I wasn't getting enough of the right kind of carbs, and I was tired a lot. But I dragged my rear end to practice and I played college basket-ball at a high level, and I was fit—I was very fit. After college, I did some running in a lot of different things, and I enjoyed ski-ing and different seasonal sports, but I didn't have the structure of the sport, of the game, of the team to keep me going in any one direction. So it was kind of sporadic and isolated incidents of, 'I'm going to hike,' or 'I'm going to run,' or things like that.

"I never could achieve that level of fitness again, and like a lot of people, I thought I was just gaining weight and becom-ing soft in all the wrong places, but I also wasn't putting in the hours working out, either. I had a life and a job and things.

"So, I found a workout called P90X. I thought, *Wow, this is something I could do because there is an actual structure to it; there's a program*. And even if there were days I couldn't do it, I could see a plan that in ninety days, I would start getting fit. And that kind of sent me on the journey of meeting people who were doing coaching with the company Beachbody."

The P90X system, as well as the Beachbody system, helped Kelli find her love of coaching and helping others. "At first I thought I would like to do this just because of the account-ability. If I'm to learn how to coach people, then I need to be fit myself, you know? Like the product of the product, I guess, and that's how I started with the coaching. I have found out that the science they are using in the workouts, the training that you see on the show *Biggest Loser* and all those kinds of things, there's the science behind it where you're maximizing the time that you're actually working out versus the mindless, endless running on the treadmill that so many of us have done."

Kelli has learned firsthand that fitness can be the Fountain of Youth for those who live the active lifestyle. "I'll tell you what," she explains, "although my body now does look much different from when I was twenty-two, I'm as fit cardiovascularly, and just as strong—or stronger—than I was in my twenties playing basketball, which I think is incredible. Never in my whole life would I have thought that was possible working out thirty to sixty minutes, five days a week."

Kelli is a firm believer in doing what you love when it comes to fitness, health, and nutrition. "When I started working out in programs that were really working, and I saw some results," she explains, "that set my desire to do it more versus, 'Peas are good for me and I should eat them, and therefore I'm going to do it.'

"That only lasts so long. So I guess I just saw the internal motivation because I just wanted to do it, but I also had the external motivation of results and feeling good, and now, of course, there's coaching."

Kelli explains that she coaches her clients with combination workouts. "All the workouts that I do are HIIT workouts, and that stands for High Intensity Interval Training. In fact, all the programs that the company Beachbody puts out are home-based ones. We do work out with people in person, but we also coach people from afar in their own workouts.

"So HIIT means high intensity interval training, and it's very interesting—if you think about somebody on a treadmill walking, and it's like *here comes a hill*, and you kick it for the stair climber or treadmill, and the incline happens for about a minute, and then you come back down and walk, right? HIIT workouts in essence are exactly the opposite of that.

"You are having prolonged exertions of energy with short bursts of rest, if you will. And that is where the fat-burning magic comes in. And that's why these workouts can truly guarantee that in thirty days you'll get ripped, and I mean, it's intense, but you're going that whole time with little bursts of rest. HIIT also can be done in sixty days or ninety days. They're all geared toward that."

Kelli is very devoted to her coaching clients who, she says, are "thirty- to forty-somethings, usually women who are busy; they're on a budget, but they want to find their mojo for the first time or regain it. They have kind of a 'bring it' mentality within themselves, and that is to say, life is crazy, it's busy, it's fast, career, kids, career, whatever.

"Everything is kind of swirling around, but they're realizing that they're not getting any more energetic as they get older, they're not getting any more fit, and they're even starting to realize that, gosh, middle age is coming up. And then sometimes, some of us, too, are looking at our parents' health issues, and that's kind of scary. And they're thinking, *What can I do?* It's amazing too, because I love it when people are like, 'So, you're able to achieve,' whatever it is I've achieved here, and 'in 'x' amount of minutes a day?'

"And I'm like, 'Yes, and you can too.' It's not, this is not like being a gym rat where you hang out there, and you leave your kids at home by themselves for hours on end, or whatever weird thing. Or, you're just married to some sort of gym, or even necessarily have to pay hundreds and hundreds of dollars every month to do this. This really can be achieved, and I can show you how. I would love to show you how, because you don't have to just believe that you're going to get more out of shape, and more tired, and drink more gallons of coffee as you get older, because you're just dragging yourself out of bed. That's what people think, typically women at a jewelry party or at a Tupperware party, and I'm like, 'Yeah I can totally show you how to do this.' And there's no magic to it. I feel like I figured the secret out and I want to share it with them, too."

Kelli is equally passionate about the Shakeology program because, she says, "For me, it is my supplement; it is all my vitamins. I am one of those people that you saw at Costco that loaded up my cart with vitamins that I just stuck in a drawer because I never used them. I couldn't remember to take them, or they hurt my tummy, or I was burping vitamins until 10:30, or whenever. So to me it's an all–in-one supplement which, depending on your exertion, is a snack or meal.

"And for people who particularly need to really shed some pounds—I mean, I don't use it as a weight-loss thing, but if they need to jumpstart their program—I do suggest Shakeology, which is, depending on how you buy it, ninety to a hundred twenty dollars a month, so that's three or four dollars a serving or meal or whatever you want to call it. But that's if they want to do Shakeology, and I mean I'll coach anybody. I still coach people who haven't even purchased anything through my business. I just want help people out."

Now it's time for Kelli to share her own top 12 tips for getting and staying fit.

Top 12 Tips from Kelli

#1: If you fall off the wagon, get right back on it. Don't just go, "Oh I messed up for today; now I can't do it at all." Instead, have the ability to say, "All right, everyone has downtimes, so let's get back into it!"

#2: Stick with it, and it will become a lifestyle. My experience is that the people who hang in there figure out a way to push themselves. That could mean doubling back after the holidays and redoing a workout that they had started and stopped. And those people push, but they also jump back in.

#3: Get addicted to the lifestyle, not the fitness. Another way of saying this is that it's a lifestyle for them; it is not something they're doing. Is nothing that they're picking up and adopting; this is what they've become. And this is what's contagious for people.

#4: Plan to succeed … with a successful plan. Have a time of day and some sort of system in place so that you know where you're going.

#5: Sometimes you just have to step it up a notch. If you're really interested in fat-burning muscle-building activities, you're going to have to push yourself more than that, because you're not actually going to burn a lot of calories.

#6: You can find the time if you make the time. In the spirit of how they say real estate is all about location, location, location, I'm going to say that the biggest excuse I hear is, "I have no time, I have no time, I have no time." What that means is that they haven't prioritized the time. They are fearful of doing, of starting, and feeling, and so they say they don't have time. They really are very pressed for time, and they simply don't know how to maximize the time that they have because they don't know what to do.

#7: Fitness shouldn't take forever. A lot of times people are very busy and they think they don't have time because they don't have an hour, or something like that. And they don't realize that there are things they can do that are less than an hour that could be effective.

#8: Get on Shakeology. Shakeology is a snack or meal replacement that can give you the nutrients your body needs to release a lot of fat.

#9: Practice more portion control. Start eating your meals using a salad plate!

#10: Move more. Find something you enjoy doing that's a physical activity and do it for at least ten minutes a day. Be active for at least ten minutes a day. Do something: walk your dog or ride your bike down the block with your kids.

#11: Eat more real food. Stop eating processed foods, engineered food, additives, and preservatives. Skip all the fast, on-the-go, eating in your car.

#12: Find something that you love to do. You will keep doing it if you love it. If you don't love it, don't do it; otherwise, you will equate exercise and fitness with misery and duty, and that's not a good combination for a lifetime. Find something that you love to do and do it, and then maybe there's specific training things that you will find that you need to do in order to be stronger at it.

Thanks, Kelli, for taking the time to speak with us and to help us achieve a better body like yours!

Chapter 12

Confuse Your Muscles
with **Donovan Green**

*"Life, money, kids, the wife, the husband, life events … at the
end of the day, these are really just excuses. The only excuse
you have to not work out is you're dead; that's it."*
~ Donovan Green

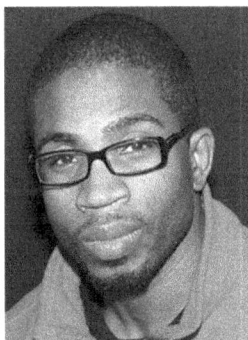

With over twelve years of professional experience, Donovan Green is known as a specialist of muscle confusion. He fuses exercises ranging from sports conditioning to yoga within one session. He is a certified personal trainer with ACE (American Council on Exercise), Nike Sparq trainer, HFTN elite coach, health counselor from the School of Integrative Nutrition, and a martial arts enthusiast.

While understanding that life can sometimes be very demanding, Donovan never allows his clients to give up on themselves or on him. He uses positive and powerful phrases as great reinforcement tools, such as, "The words 'I can't' do not exist." He is passionate about helping others achieve greatness physically as well as mentally and spiritually. His approach to good health is based on the overall wellness of each individual through a more holistic standpoint.

Donovan has a very diverse list of clients who are devoted to his unique style of training and are passionate about maintaining their physical appearance, including celebrities such as Dr. Oz. His energy embodies greatness and empowers his clients to attain their specific goals. He strongly believes that procrastination is the key to failure.

Donovan works for LA Boxing in Norwalk, Connecticut, and even though fitness is clearly his passion, he considers himself primarily a life coach. Like many trainers who wind up in the fields of health, fitness, and lifestyle, Donovan's struggle with his own physicality began in childhood.

"I was a chubby kid," he explains. "I was a fat kid, and my aunt would always tease me. She'd say, 'You got man boobs,' 'You got a big belly, 'Pull your stomach in,' and all these things, and it was not a hurtful thing for me as a kid growing up; it was a fun gesture. But as I got older, when I hit thirteen years old, I got into fitness with my uncle, who had a gym downstairs in his apartment."

Donovan credits martial arts, among other things, for fueling his interest in fitness. "I started watching a lot of martial arts movies like Kung Fu stuff on Channel 5 on Saturdays," he explains. "I started to actually study the martial arts. So, I realized I had a love for martial arts; I started reaching out and getting more involved in nutrition. My mind was much more clear and my energy was up."

While physical fitness and nutrition had his attention, it would be a few years and a few occupations before it had his full-time job status. Donovan recalls, "I got into different occupations. I was a barber for over fifteen years, I learned carpentry, I learned electrical work, plumbing, but during all of those times when I was growing up and doing all these different things, I was still doing fitness.

"I was still talking to people about exercise, and trying to get my friends to work out, and going to the gym, and doing all this intricate stuff in fitness. And I used to always hear, 'D, you need to start working out. You need to start getting people working out. Do it as a profession. Become a trainer.' It hit me one day, and I decided to be a trainer, and that's what brought me here many years later."

Muscle confusion is a big part of what has made Donovan so fit and so successful as a fitness trainer to this day. "I am a big believer in muscle confusion," he says. "So I have moments where I do a lot of body building style workouts, and then I do more on the high-intensity training interval drills. I'll do full martial arts training. I studied Krav Maga, which is an Israeli military method of doing martial arts. I would do a full circuit of that. I am always changing it up. I don't really have one specific program. I'll do yoga or Pilates. So I'll mix it up. I always keep my body moving, always guessing *What's next*?"

Donovan has one of the most original answers of all time when it comes to who would be his dream trainer. "God would be my dream trainer," he insists. "I would love to sit down with him and get all the knowledge he could give me. I don't want to train with him for a long time, just one hour. I don't want to know about world peace or anything like that. I want to know about the secrets of fitness. You need a whole power hour. Just give me all the knowledge you've got, God, right now, and I'll only take the hour. I won't take the whole world—just one hour. And that's my honest answer."

Donovan personally trains, be it in a classroom setting or individually, over seventy clients every week. He does muscle confusion training with his clients as well. "They never know what they are going to get," he explains, "so they love to hate and hate to love me at the same time. I will implement kickboxing one day, and the next day it'll be kettle bells. Then we'll do boxing, and then only weight training. I am always intriguing their mind. Always making them not get used to anything, but at the end of the day, it's always hard, no matter what their level is.

"So, if somebody is a beginner, I am going to give them something hard for a beginner. Like, if somebody's a beginner, I am not going to tell them to give me fifty push-ups, I am going to tell them to give me ten. That's hard for them. If someone is extremely overweight, I am going to ask him or her to sit down and get up ten times. That's hard for them, but I want them to learn that this is a game. It's where failure is what you are looking for, and fitness is the only thing in life where failure is the key. When you fail in fitness, and your muscles give up on you, that is a good thing. That is not a bad thing. And they understand that. Go for failure. Go to where your body says, 'Oh my God.'"

When it comes to putting his clients through the paces, Donovan offers them a veritable buffet of options. "I implement a whole bunch of different stuff," he says of his clients' personalized workouts. "I don't use strategies, because everyone has that. Everyone has strategies, and everyone says, 'Do cardio before you work out, do cardio after you work out.' I apply the same scenario, the same method, as I would for food: 'Eat when hungry, drink when thirsty.' I give them a basic, simple guideline on what they should be doing, and it is up to them to implement what works for them.

"Because I cannot tell somebody, 'Do cardio this time, do cardio that time,' because it might not work for them. Their body type might not respond at that particular time of the day. So I will give them a list of different things so that they have choices to make. And I give them all the facts from all the years of research of what I have seen and what I have learned and what I witnessed and what I know. And then they'll take that information and follow through with it."

For those who can't quite afford a personal trainer, or even a membership to their local gym, Donovan is all too happy to offer several tips for saving money. "One of the main things," he insists, is to "use what you have at home, especially if you have stairs. Stairs are like the best equipment you can use for cardio, so much better than a six-thousand-dollar machine in the gym.

"You have your spouse, or you can work out with a partner. Use what you have around you in your house. Look around and see what you can lift, or what you can push. Or, go to the gym and do team packages with a trainer. It is a great way to save money."

Donovan insists that the key to a sustainable workout isn't in what you do or even who trains you, but in whether or not you're ready to commit to a brand new lifestyle. "They commit to it," he says of people who crave a better body and are finally ready to do something about it. "And they commit to me as their trainer. They will alleviate or eliminate things out of their lives, that extra expense, and look at me as the important part of their day, and they will commit."

Now comes the portion I always get the most excited about. In the next section, you will find Donovan's top 12 tips for getting and keeping a better body.

Top 12 Tips from Donovan

#1: Timing is everything. It is about commitment; there are people who don't commit well, and there are people who do commit. People have come to a place in life where they say, "No more; it's time to change." And they don't just say it; they actually act on it, and they decide to commit to someone who's going to hold them accountable.

#2: Take a break, but not too big a break! The people who don't work out when they go on vacation never really experience real results. They don't know what they gain, so they have nothing to lose. The people who experience real results work really hard for what they're gaining, and they don't want to lose what they've gained. So when they go on vacation, they will indulge in certain foods, and to me that is awesome. Please, go on your vacation and enjoy your food. But they also understand: you still have to work out.

#3: Be wary of gym memberships. They offer you all these crazy deals for no reason. Please … you're not even going to use the gym on a regular basis, and you are only going to go there for twenty minutes, an hour at the most, if that. But gym memberships are traps that people fall for.

#4: Get on YouTube! Everything is on YouTube. Type in anything you want to, and YouTube will give you lots of ideas about how to keep your workouts fresh. There are trainers all over YouTube who are looking for exposure, and they're giving people all this free information and real information, not just fabricated advice.

#5: Quit making excuses. Life, money, kids, the wife, the husband, life events … at the end of the day, these are really just excuses. The only excuse you have not to work out is you're dead; that's it.

#6: Get your focus back. I tell my clients to Google the amount of people who die every year from high blood pressure and diabetes. Thousands of people die every day from complications of stroke. I also tell them to type the word funerals into a search engine, and look at the funerals of the people who died today. Look at gravestones. I don't pretty things up for people; I don't give them the pretty picture. I don't let them focus on what they look like, and whether they have a tight butt or a good-looking chest. I don't focus on that. I focus on a healthy lifestyle, and on being healthy. And once you reach them, they bring their butts right back to the gym, because no one really wants to die, especially when they can do something about it.

#7: Ban the television. Get rid of the television in the house. Get rid of cable, period. Get rid of it.

#8: Create a healthy shopping list. Stick to the shopping list, and make sure it's reasonable and realistic. So if you like Oreo cookies, by all means, put Oreo cookies on your shopping list. But don't go crazy and put all of your cookies and ice cream and cake batter and Chips Ahoy.

#9: Watch less TV. Every time you turn that TV on—especially if you're watching the news—you are exposed to negative stuff. It shocks your nerves; it shocks your mind. That adds to stress. Four days without TV, you don't realize it at first, but you actually do better.

#10: Spend more time together. Take a walk with your family instead of a drive. You get to spend quality time with your family; you get to talk more; you get to build more; and you get to know each other more. Even I am guilty of this: I'm in a room on the computer, my son is up in his room, all the time now; my wife is in her room; my baby, he's in his room doing stuff, watching *Dora*. But quality family time is important and essential for brainpower and motivation. When you spend more time together with your family, it motivates you to want to be healthier, and you want to be around them for a longer time. So you do everything in your power to be healthier, to be around the kids and to grow up with them. If you live in a household where everything is perfect, and everybody is lying to everybody— after a while you don't even care about being around those people, or even living that long. It's kinda weird, but that's just how people think. Having a bond with others kind of gives a more powerful "why" to working out.

#11: It's not all physical. We're all rich in our own ways, and we need to embrace that wealth. That wealth comes from spirituality, friendships, being able to get up and look outside, having the luxury of the use of our legs and arms, and enjoying the access to simple things like hot and cold running water. We need to embrace ourselves as humans.

#12: No more excuses. Stop making excuses! At the end of the day, you are just full of … it. Excuses lead you to nothing but the pits—the dumps.

Donovan is a true inspiration, and I hope these tips have inspired you as much as they've inspired me!

Appendix

- Top 12 Tips from All 12 Trainers

- Top 12 Habits That Keep You Working Out for the Long Haul

- Top 12 Excuses

- Top 12: What *Really* Holds People Back

- Top 12 Fitness Traps

- Top 12 Free and Simple Changes to Save Your Life

- Trainers' Top 12 Dream Trainers

- Trainers' Top 12 Dream Clients

Top 12 Tips from All 12 Trainers

Top 12 Tips from Adriana Martin

#1: Find a workout that's right for you!

#2: Timing is everything.

#3: Less is more.

#4: Money shouldn't be an obstacle.

#5: Invest in food!

#6: Have a sustainable workout.

#7: Have realistic expectations.

#8: Build a memory bank instead of an excuse bank!

#9: Do it for more than your looks!

#10: Stop making excuses.

#11: Forget your genetics.

#12: Believe in yourself!

Top 12 Tips from Ally Shumate

#1: Balance your cardio.

#2: Lose your all-or-nothing mentality.

#3: Don't let your life get in the way.

#4: Little things can really add up.

#5: Get rid of the fear.

#6: Walk more.

#7: Stand up more.

#8: Sometimes, less really IS more.

#9: Muscle is where it's at.

#10: Not all food is created equal.

#11: Eat five times a day.

#12: Fruits are fine, but veggies are divine.

Top 12 Tips from Ashley Borden

#1: Plan to succeed.

#2: See the bigger picture.

#3: Don't do everything; do something.

#4: Layer your goals.

#5: Stay positive.

#6: Don't go it alone.

#7: Try something new.

#8: Choose your environment carefully.

#9: Don't be intimidated.

#10: Dig deeper.

#11: Hydrate yourself.

#12: Lose the soda.

Top 12 Tips from David Vaughan

#1: Make lifestyle choices that are easy to maintain.

#2: It's okay to take a break—just not indefinitely.

#3: Avoid stress eating.

#4: Eat less, do more—period.

#5: Choose your food wisely.

#6: Watch your sodium.

#7: Count ALL your calories.

#8: Finding the right fit with your trainer is key.

#9: Find a trainer who appreciates flexibility.

#10: Find a trainer who listens.

#11: Be in it to win it.

#12: Don't underestimate the power of fun!

Top 12 Tips from Franklin Antoian

#1: Get a workout program that fits you.

#2: Mix it up every three months.

#3: Take a vacation from exercise.

#4: Avoid doing too much too soon.

#5: Don't set such huge goals for yourself right away.

#6: Give yourself ten minutes.

#7: Avoid the world's top three excuses for not working out!

#8: Exercise can be fun.

#9: You don't have to walk much, but walk every day.

#10: Show some resistance.

#11: Stretch for your health.

#12: Control what you can control.

Top 12 Tips from Gilad Janklowicz

#1: To stay inspired, find a workout you can sustain.

#2: Don't make contracts in your mind that your body can't keep.

#3: Don't give it all away.

#4: Slow and steady wins the race.

#5: Don't use the people on TV as your role model.

#6: Sweat is good for you!

#7: Beware of abundance.

#8: Make fitness a priority.

#9: Maintain your machine.

#10: Be proud of what's in your fridge!

#11: It just takes a little bit of control.

#12: Decide to decide, then do something about it!

Top 12 Tips from Heather Hodges

#1: It's okay to have fun when you're exercising.

#2: Don't do too much at once.

#3: Avoid the trap of overtraining.

#4: Your body needs rest.

#5: Don't let being a mom limit you from being all that you can be.

#6: Stop buying bigger clothes.

#7: Skip the sugar.

#8: Start small, but start somewhere.

#9: Go outside and play.

#10: Family first.

#11: Patient, heal thyself.

#12: Don't neglect the spiritual aspect of why we train.

APPENDIX

Top 12 Tips from Lindsay Wright

#1: Don't do too much too soon.

#2: Rest is critical.

#3: Breaks can be beneficial.

#4: Find your niche, and the passion will follow.

#5: Pick the right kind of class for you.

#6: Take your injuries seriously.

#7: Get hydrated.

#8: Start a weight-lifting program.

#9: Build movement into your day.

#10: Remember that exercise and getting fit are so much more mental than physical.

#11: Find a trainer who inspires you.

#12: Just get started.

Top 12 Tips from Doc Masters

#1: Fitness takes time.

#2: You are who you hang around with.

#3: Don't eat anything that's in a box.

#4: You have to stay away from high fructose corn syrup.

#5: You have to stay away from artificial sweeteners like aspartame.

#6: Stay away from table salt.

#7: Kosher is kosher.

#8: Chlorine is a poison.

#9: Stop drinking bottled water!

#10: Don't try to get fit in a week.

#11: All change is good.

#12: By learning, we teach. By teaching, we learn.

Top 12 Tips from Tamilee Webb

#1: Do what's right for you.

#2: Fight boredom.

#3: You can make diets work, if you do the work—and stick with them.

#4: If you don't make time for health and fitness now, you will make time for illness later.

#5: Listen to your body. (It listens to you!)

#6: A little means a lot.

#7: Start with a positive affirmation.

#8: Educate yourself.

#9: Your body is meant to move.

#10: Give yourself 84 days.

#11: Know your goals.

#12: Find a good fit with your trainer.

Top 12 Tips from Kelli Buzzard

#1: If you fall off the wagon, get right back on it.

#2: Stick with it, and it will become a lifestyle.

#3: Get addicted to the lifestyle, not the fitness.

#4: Plan to succeed with a successful plan.

#5: Sometimes you just have to step it up a notch.

#6: You can find the time if you make the time.

#7: Fitness shouldn't take forever.

#8: Get on Shakeology.

#9: Practice more portion control.

#10: Move more.

#11: Eat more real food.

#12: Find something that you love to do.

Top 12 Tips from Donovan Green

#1: Timing is everything.

#2: Take a break, but not too big a break!

#3: Be wary of gym memberships

#4: Get on YouTube!

#5: Quit making excuses.

#6: Get your focus back.

#7: Ban the television.

#8: Create a healthy shopping list.

#9: Watch less TV.

#10: Spend more time together.

#11: It's not all physical.

#12: No more excuses.

Top 12 Habits That Keep You Working Out for the Long Haul

I asked each trainer about sustainable workout patterns: what sets apart someone who works out long term from others who burn out? Here are the top answers:

#1: Your body doesn't know the difference between being at the gym or being at home. Workout anywhere! (Adriana)

#2: Working out is a lifestyle—not something you do for the short term. (Tamilee)

#3: Figure out a way to push yourself—whatever that means to you. (Kelli)

#4: Schedule three workouts per week. Don't overwhelm yourself with an over-the-top workout schedule. (Lindsay)

#5: Get a really good, hard workout in thirty to forty-five minutes, working your whole body, two to three days per week. Three days would be max. (Ally)

#6: Every week make your plan for the following week, and keep that plan in front of you all the time. Plan the work(out), and work the plan. (Ashley)

#7: Make measurable long-term and short-term goals. (David)

#8: What's going to make you stay fit is to have recreational activities that you like to do. (Doc)

#9: Commit and be accountable. Commit to a trainer if you can, but commit to someone. (Donovan)

#10: Do this for your own benefit and your own health and fitness by keeping a program that you can do with ease. You should be sore, but you should feel successful and should not be over-the-top tired. (Gilad)

#11: Once you get a workout program, design it around your goals and your schedule. (Franklin)

#12: Begin with a mission; understand what motivates you to start working out in the first place, and then remember that. (Heather)

Top 12 Excuses

I asked each trainer to think of someone he or she has tried to persuade to work out for a long time, but just can't get this person to exercise. When asked what reasons these people give for not working out, here are the top answers:

#1: Time; I don't have the time. (Allyson, Donovan, Ashley, Franklin, David, Heather, Kelli, Adriana, Lindsay)

#2: I'm too tired; I just don't have the energy. (Allyson, David)

#3: I just can't get around to it. (Allyson)

#4: I don't really need to; I'm just not interested. (Donovan, Ashley, Gilad, Heather)

#5: I don't know what to do. (Franklin)

#6: I don't like gyms. (Franklin)

#7: I have health issues that limit exercise. (Gilad)

#8: Healthy food doesn't taste good. (Gilad)

#9: I don't like to sweat. (Gilad)

#10: I feel like I'm too old. (David)

#11: I need to find childcare. (Heather)

APPENDIX

#12: Money; I can't afford it. (Adriana)

BONUS: I'm genetically predisposed to be overweight. (Adriana)

139

Top 12: What Really Holds People Back

Each trainer shared the main excuses people use to avoid working out, then they were asked what they think really holds those people back. Here are the top answers:

#1: Fear they won't be successful (Allyson, Kelli)

#2: Lack of convenience (Donovan)

#3: Intimidated by working out in front of other people (Ashley)

#4: Misinformation or lack of information (Franklin)

#5: Self-destruction (Donovan, Gilad)

#6: Overwhelmed by the need to lose so much weight (David)

#7: Lack of activity breeds lack of energy. (David)

#8: Not a big enough reason why (Heather)

#9: Discouraged by no early success (Kelli)

#10: Don't believe in themselves (Adriana)

#11: Taking that first step is hard. (Lindsay)

#12: It is tough to break deep-seeded bad eating habits. (Lindsay)

Top 12 Fitness Traps

I asked each trainer, "What fitness traps do people fall into when getting started on an exercise program?" Here are the top answers:

#1: Focus too much on cardio. (Allyson)

#2: All-or-nothing mentality (Allyson, Ashley)

#3: People try to do too much too soon. (Doc, Franklin, Gilad, David, Heather, Lindsay)

#4: Unreasonable expectations from infomercials, gym memberships, quick-and-easy diet products, and reality television shows (Donovan, Gilad, Adriana)

#5: Unreasonable eating or fad diets (David)

#6: No plan (Kelli)

#7: Doing the same thing over and over again—not mixing up the workout. (Kelli)

#8: Expecting unreasonable results too soon. If it took years to put on a lot of weight, give yourself some time to take it off. (Gilad, Adriana)

#9: Forgetting the good stuff—so write it down or remember it. (Ashley, Adriana)

#10: Not finding a workout that is fun (Lindsay)

#11: People blame and are hard on themselves. (Adriana)

#12: Boredom; not having the next phase of working out to
   look forward to. (Ashley)

Top 12 Free and Simple Changes to Save Your Life

I asked each trainer, "If you were boss of the world and could force people to make three free, simple changes that would improve their health, what would those changes be?" Here are the top answers:

#1: Walk more, and walk to places. (Allyson, Donovan, Franklin)

#2: Stand up more; move around more. (Allyson, Gilad, David, Adriana, Lindsay)

#3: Get your core strong. (Allyson)

#4: Drink more water. (Doc, Ashley, Lindsay)

#5: Get your exercise through play. Find things you like to do that are ACTIVE. (Kelli)

#6: Make a healthy shopping list. Eat real foods. Some individual tips: Don't eat anything from a box; eat more fruit; eat more vegetables; don't drink soda; don't eat table salt. (Doc, Donovan, Adriana, Ashley)

#7: Get rid of the television (or at least cable). (Donovan)

#8: Spend more time with the family; play more; eat dinner together. (Donovan, Gilad, Heather)

#9: Learn how to read food labels and then do it. (David)

#10: Do more strength training. (Franklin, Lindsay)

#11: Stretch every day, or roll out. (Ashley, Franklin)

#12: Use smaller plates; eat less. (Gilad, David, Kelli)

Trainers' Top 12 Dream Trainers

I asked each trainer, "Who would be your dream trainer if you were the client?" Here are the top answers:

#1: Rachel Cosgrove (Allyson)

#2: God (Donovan)

#3: Karl List (Ashley)

#4: Jennifer Aniston (Franklin)

#5: Elaria (Gilad)

#6: Steve at Equinox, New York (Gilad)

#7: Jillian Michaels (David)

#8: Dara Torres (Heather)

#9: Shaun Thompson (Kelli)

#10: Brett Hoebel (Kelli)

#11: Deepak Chopra (Adriana)

#12: Bob Harper (Lindsay Wright)

Trainers' Top 12 Dream Clients

I asked each trainer, "Who would be your dream client?" Here are the top answers:

#1: Kobe Bryant (Doc)

#2: Ryan Scheckler (Doc)

#3: L.L. Cool J (Donovan)

#4: Tyra Banks (Ashley)

#5: Jennifer Aniston (Franklin)

#6: Charlize Theron (Gilad)

#7: Dana White (David)

#8: Charles Barkley (Heather)

#9: Average people (Ally, Kelli)

#10: Hugh Jackman (Lindsay Wright)

#11: Anthony Robbins (Adriana)

#12: Miranda Lambert (Tamilee)

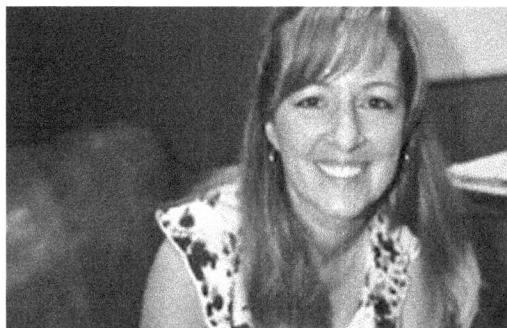

About the Author

Tiffany Youngren, founder of TransferofHealth.com

Tiffany Youngren is the founder and CEO of www. TransferofHealth.com, a website-slash-blog featuring recipes, wellness tips, fitness articles, and more, which she started in 2011. In the process of researching food and exercise for her own family's wellness, and to develop TransferofHealth.com, she has met and developed relationships with countless bloggers, dietitians, foodies, naturopaths, and other health and wellness professionals, as well as fitness experts.

Tiffany and her husband of over twenty years, Duane, have three (nearly) grown children. Both grew up in scenic Skagit County in Northwest Washington, where they sold real estate for over eighteen years. Tiffany was active in the community, business organizations, and her church, where she sang with several of the worship teams at Christ the King Community Church locations in Northwest Washington. She moved to Austin, Texas, with her family in 2008, then to Columbus,

Montana, in 2012. She continues to thrive in the business world where she assists entrepreneurs, management, and employees in a variety of industries including real estate and finance. You can see what Tiffany is working on now by visiting her LinkedIn profile at www.linkedin.com/in/tiffanyyoungren/.

Tiffany has always loved to cook, and considers herself a huge foodie. Nutrition has been an interest of Tiffany's for some time, and she has an innate fondness for physical fitness. She was an athlete in high school, and enjoyed sampling many of the workouts featured in her new book, *Better Body Wannabe*, including P90X, yoga, pilates, and Zumba.

Fitness has also played a big role in Tiffany's interest in health and longevity. Like readers of her book, Tiffany struggles with making time to work out—and talking herself into doing it when she does have time. Compiling the trainers' interviews for *Better Body Wannabe* has allowed her to see that fitness is a lifestyle, not an event—a truly encouraging thought! She sincerely hopes the book encourages others as well.

www.ingramcontent.com/pod-product-compliance
Lightning Source LLC
Chambersburg PA
CBHW070840300326
41935CB00038B/1161